Springer Series on Child and Family Studies

Series Editor
Nirbhay N. Singh
Medical College of Georgia
Augusta University
Augusta, Georgia, USA

More information about this series at http://www.springer.com/series/13095

Laura Nabors

Medical and Mental Health During Childhood

Psychosocial Perspectives
and Positive Outcomes

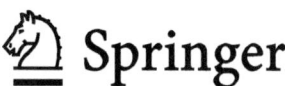 Springer

Laura Nabors
School of Human Services
University of Cincinnati
Cincinnati, OH, USA

Springer Series on Child and Family Studies
ISBN 978-3-319-31115-9   ISBN 978-3-319-31117-3   (eBook)
DOI 10.1007/978-3-319-31117-3

Library of Congress Control Number: 2016939666

© Springer International Publishing Switzerland 2016
This work is subject to copyright. All rights are reserved by the Publisher, whether the whole or part of the material is concerned, specifically the rights of translation, reprinting, reuse of illustrations, recitation, broadcasting, reproduction on microfilms or in any other physical way, and transmission or information storage and retrieval, electronic adaptation, computer software, or by similar or dissimilar methodology now known or hereafter developed.
The use of general descriptive names, registered names, trademarks, service marks, etc. in this publication does not imply, even in the absence of a specific statement, that such names are exempt from the relevant protective laws and regulations and therefore free for general use.
The publisher, the authors and the editors are safe to assume that the advice and information in this book are believed to be true and accurate at the date of publication. Neither the publisher nor the authors or the editors give a warranty, express or implied, with respect to the material contained herein or for any errors or omissions that may have been made.

Printed on acid-free paper

This Springer imprint is published by Springer Nature
The registered company is Springer International Publishing AG Switzerland

Thanks to my family

Preface

This textbook is designed to provide information for those interested in improving their understanding of childhood health and mental health problems. The goal of each chapter is to address a childhood medical or mental health issue and share knowledge about diagnosing the problem, understanding psychosocial issues faced by children coping with the problem, and developing a framework of ways to improve child functioning. The overall goal of this book is to discuss and learn about evidence-based treatments and review ideas for interventions. Opening chapters review several medical conditions, including asthma, diabetes, and cancer. Because coping with pain is a common issue for children with these medical conditions, a chapter is devoted to discussing ways to assist children in coping with pain related to medical conditions (e.g., medical procedures). In addition, this chapter also addresses coping with medical fears. Medical fears are an important issue to highlight, because treatment may become a difficult experience for children. In this textbook, I also address mental health problems for children, including autism spectrum disorders, anxiety, depression, conduct disorders, and attention-deficit/hyperactivity disorder. At the close of this book, my hope is that you will be well versed in evidence-based interventions for children with the aforementioned problems and have an understanding of how to identify health and mental health problems and intervene to assist children in moving forward in a positive developmental trajectory.

Chapters in this textbook are organized into two parts. The first part of each chapter presents new information about diagnosing the problem and treating the child to maximize positive development. Subsequent sections present an in-depth view of psychosocial issues, review key information in the evidence base, discuss practical ideas for treatment, and present a case study. Cases depicted in this book are not "real," but were developed based on a recollection of my real-world cases from 20 years in the field. The final sections are a summary, which present key concepts and contain exercises to review fundamental information in the chapter.

My perspective is developmental in nature. It is important to recognize the breadth of change and growth for children from birth through adulthood. A developmental perspective assesses child functioning and adjustment throughout the child's development from birth through the early adult years. In other words, this perspective encourages assessment and study of the individual throughout his or her life course—from infancy to old age. Coming from a developmental perspective, we are concerned with age and how it might impact an individual's adjustment. To address all the literature at all the key developmental phases—toddlerhood, preschool age, elementary school, middle school, and high school—is beyond the scope of this book. Thus, discussion in chapters will primarily focus on elementary school years. The elementary school years are a key period for prevention and intervention efforts that may lead to lasting change for the child that will influence his or her development in a positive manner.

In addition to a developmental perspective, I was heavily influenced by the idea that "context is important." To that end, I agree with the "systems perspective," perhaps, most by that espoused by Urie Bronfenbrenner (1989) in his *Ecological Systems Theory*. The child is "set," if you will, in contexts and the critical contexts for the elementary school-age child are family and school. I will discuss these contexts in depth in chapters of this book. Further research is needed to address child functioning in other contexts such as neighborhood, after-school, and extracurricular settings. Hopefully, you will be encouraged to conduct new research in these key areas.

I was also strongly influenced by my professors in graduate school. They encouraged their students to understand the science and facts presented in literature focusing on children and then to try to make the knowledge we had gained "work" to help a child. I began to believe in the contribution of research when one of my mentors stated that one can help more children with good research, because they can be a bit more confident when they have current knowledge of what works for whom. One of the best recommendations for reading the literature is to use it to find ideas to support one's treatment efforts to make a positive difference in the lives of children and families. Taking a deep dive into the literature to understand how to improve child self-esteem, quality of life, and functioning is invaluable. The literature will also illuminate ways to reduce the impact of negative factors shaping the child's developmental trajectory.

Another influence on my view of treatment of children came from what I have learned from my parents. Both are clinicians who are interested in improving the well-being of their patients. They focus on the positive and how to move their patients forward. A functional analysis of behavior will help us understand what factors trigger (or cause) positive behaviors, maintain them, and improve them. A functional analysis of behavior considers the triggering factors for a behavior, what rewards or reinforces a behavior, and what could possibly maintain or change a behavior. The next step is observing the child—in a case study approach—to see what works. When interventions are successful, we can then maximize "best treatment" for the patient. Therefore, in the sections within chapters that discuss intervening with children, I will reflect on ideas from the literature and from case studies to explain what is going on with a child. Interventions to help children cope with particular problems will also be illustrated.

Being positive brings more benefits to clients and strengthens their self-esteem. This orientation is reflected in the chapters by emphasizing understanding psychosocial factors and environmental factors that will promote resilience for the child and his or her family. It is my belief that the promotion of child strengths and use of interventions to decrease stressors for the child and family will improve quality of life and, ultimately, health outcomes for children with medical and mental health conditions. Applied studies, or studies in the field, can provide many ideas for promoting the growth of children and families. Moreover, monitoring the progress of each client or patient, to determine if assets are being maximized and positive functioning is being increased, may be associated with best practices in clinical care.

In closing, I want to thank you for reading this book and I hope you enjoy learning about ways to help children.

Cincinnati, OH   Laura Nabors

Reference

Bronfenbrenner, U. (1989). Ecological systems theory. *Annals of Child Development, 6,* 187–249.

Contents

About the Author

Laura Nabors, Ph.D. is an associate professor in the Health Promotion and Education Program, in the School of Human Services, in the College of Education, Criminal Justice, and Human Services, at the University of Cincinnati. She is also a diplomat in clinical child and adolescent psychology for the American Board of Professional Psychology. Dr. Nabors graduated with a doctorate in clinical psychology, with a focus on working with children and families, from the University of Memphis. She has interests in children's health and mental health issues and helping children with these issues to become integrated into their schools and activities. She is concerned with wellness and promoting adaptation for children and their families, especially in community settings.

Chapter 1
Introduction

Introduction

This chapter provides key information about helping a child with a health or mental health problem in schools. The role of a health educator is defined for the reader, so that the reader can understand the breadth of professionals associated with this term. Schools are the primary setting for young children. Therefore, policy and planning for them in this setting is critical to review so that health educators have an idea of what types of programming will need to be implemented to help children achieve to the best of their abilities. Consequently, Section 504 plans and Individual Education Programs are reviewed in order to provide background to help readers understand ways to record care plans in order for children with special health and mental health needs can have their needs met at school. Special programming in school also ensures that their progress will be tracked annually and this allows school staff and educators to make sure that children are keeping pace with peers in terms of academic, social, and emotional development.

Definition of Health Educator. This book was developed for health educators. A health educator is defined as any health professional that plays a key role in educating children and parents about a child health or mental health issues. This would encompass students in health education, psychology, social work, medicine, and nursing. The health educator also delivers education to assist the child and caregiver or parent in learning more about the child's medical or mental health condition. This education could be disease specific or designed to provide knowledge that would enhance child psychological and social functioning.

© Springer International Publishing Switzerland 2016
L. Nabors, *Medical and Mental Health During Childhood*, Springer
Series on Child and Family Studies, DOI 10.1007/978-3-319-31117-3_1

Helping a Child with a Health or Mental Health Problem in Schools

Supporting Children with Special Health Care Needs in Schools. Children with special health care needs are at risk for poor academic performance in the school setting when their health care needs are not met (Baker, Hebbeler, Davis-Alldritt, Anderson, & Knauer, 2015). There may be a shortage of nursing staff in the schools to care for children's special health care needs. Therefore, one role for health professionals is to advocate for increased nursing staff in schools. It may be the case that one nurse is assigned to several schools, and this may be insufficient to cover health care or emergency health care needs when they arise. Furthermore, advocating for nurse "availability" in terms of ensuring there is sufficient nursing staff to cover child needs across different schools is another area for advocacy.

O'Connor, Howell-Meurs, Kvalsvig, and Goldfeld (2014) presented a comprehensive model for consideration of the needs of children with special needs in school settings. They proposed that up to 20 % of the children in schools may need special supports to function optimally. Similar to Baker et al. (2015), these authors proposed that children with special needs (or special health care needs) may not function to their full academic potential without supports. O'Connor et al. recommended taking a broad view, considering "individual, school, and family circumstances" (p. 15) when planning for academic success. Although diagnosis may be a helpful starting point for understanding a child's needs, O'Connor et al. recommended considering a child's functional abilities, which include physical abilities (movement, ability to navigate at school), social participation, academic skills, and abilities to perform "activities of daily living" (p. 18) when designing plans for children with special needs. Their model also presented school connectedness, service availability (and service needs), and family functioning as important components contributing to child functioning. Taking a comprehensive look, in multiple domains of the child's life allows the school team to determine factors influencing a child's functioning and account for these factors when developing school plans. O'Connor et al. also recommended that a multidisciplinary team develops school plans, which allows for comprehensive perspectives on meeting the child's needs in multiple domains. The multidisciplinary team is a group comprised of medical experts and those professionals needed to help the child advance his or her skills, such as the school psychologist, occupational therapist, and special educators. Their model provides a useful tool for thinking of interventions to support children with special needs in school settings.

Children with a variety of special needs, such as mental health problems and chronic medical conditions, benefit from regular assessment and evaluation to determine ways to meet their needs in the school setting in order for them to benefit from their education (Boulet, Boyle, & Schieve, 2009). Children may also need regular screenings to determine needs for assistive technology and special equipment needed to improve their classroom experiences. Some of the technology needed might include assistive communication devices or special medical equipment. Children with special needs may also be at risk for long-term complications with cognitive functioning, which can impede academic attainment. Thus, regular screening of children's cognitive abilities and academic achievement can be critical to determining a school plan that will allow them to continue advancing in terms of academics (Forrest, Bevans, Riley, Crespo, & Louis, 2011). The child's medical team needs to be involved in providing recommendations to teachers and school staff, in order to provide guidance about modifications for the child that will optimize his or her access to an appropriate educational experience. Although information about child strengths may be lacking on many educational plans, this is an important area to address. Assessment of child strengths and consideration of building upon child strengths and interests should be critical components of written educational planning for children with special health care needs (Nelson, Alexander, & Molnar, 2015).

Houtrow, Larson, Olson, Newacheck, and Halfon (2014) assessed the prevalence of children with disabilities from 2001 to 2011, performing a secondary data analysis using the National Health Interview Survey. Their results indicated that about six million children had special needs in 2011. They found that the number of children with mental health care problems and neurodevelopmental disabilities was increasing. Mills and Cunningham (2014) mentioned that educational planning for children with significant emotional programs should be developed with an eye toward using the least restrictive environment (LRE). These authors noted that children with mental health problems have a tendency to be placed outside of the classroom, especially in the cases of more severe emotional and behavioral disturbances. Mills and Cunningham reported that approximately 6.5 % of the children attending schools have mental health problems and many may have Individual Education Programs that are not in the least restrictive setting. This can be very problematic, in that most of these children have significant emotional and social delays that may be best remediated when they can interact with peers who are functioning within a normal range behaviorally, emotionally, and socially. A question then arises as to whether the needs of the children who are developing more typically can be met in a classroom setting when there are one or more children with significant mental health problems in the classroom. It is possible to develop a classroom environment to promote functioning of all youth, and health and mental health care providers need to keep in mind ideas for maximizing the growth of all children in the classroom when they are developing inclusion plans for children with special needs.

Evans, Sapia, Axelrod-Lowie, and Glomb (2002) wrote about collaboration between the mental health provider and school staff to "level" the field and develop the most effective educational plan for children with mental health problems. They emphasized the importance of developing a collaborative relationship with the special education team. Consideration of who should be involved in service provision, what services should be provided, and what types of accommodations should be made to academic work (e.g., more time to take tests) should be considered when discussing the development of individualized planning for children with mental health problems. These authors noted that the development and continual evaluation of individualized plans for children with mental health problems is a challenge, in that development takes expertise, planning, time, and funding. However, Evans et al. were in favor of developing special programming to assure the most appropriate education for a child. In fact, special education planning for a child with mental health problems can serve a protective function, especially if the child is exhibiting significant behavior problems which impede his or her academic performance. Confidentiality of specialized school planning is important and involving parents in the plan allows them to share insights about their child (Evans et al., 2002).

The Council on Children with Disabilities (2007) wrote a policy statement with guidelines for inclusion of children with chronic diseases and disabling conditions in school settings. The paper, which appears in *Pediatrics*, began with a rationale for providing special services, such as nursing care, speech and language services, and occupational therapy for youth with special needs. The rationale was that services should be provided if they improve children's access to the education they need in schools. The paper was written for physicians, but the guidelines may be beneficial for other medical professionals. In this paper, the increased stress on schools—because more children with complex needs are being served in schools—was noted, which is important because schools can be overwhelmed by a child's medical or mental health needs and appropriate support from the child's medical team can make "the difference" in helping school staff to include a child with health or mental health needs in regular education settings. In cases of children with significant health needs, it may be necessary to have both an educational and special health care plan. Another goal for the medical team is to be aware of the family's preferences for the child and to balance family wishes with the school's capabilities. Balancing family and school concerns, and ensuring that family or parent wishes are met, is an important goal when developing school planning for the child.

Individual Education Programs. Halfon, Houtrow, Larson, and Newacheck (2012) stated that having a chronic condition is a heavy burden for children, restricting their activities and involvement in the school setting. An Individualized Education Program (IEP) is a written statement developed to address the special needs of a child with a chronic condition or disability in the school setting (Individuals with Disabilities Education Act, 2004). Children and adolescents between 3 and 21 years of age with specifically identified special needs or disabilities are eligible for special education services and IEPs (Osborne & Russo, 2014). Parent permission is needed for assessment of the child's abilities and to develop an IEP. Steps that occur before plan development include identification of the child and referral for evaluation by experts—professionals with expertise in the areas where special services may be needed. After initial screening and assessment of child needs, members of the special education team meet to develop a written plan to meet the child's educational needs in the most appropriate manner in the least restrictive setting. Annual updates to the plan are required (annual evaluation meetings are held) and every 3 years a re-assessment of the child's skills is required to update the plan. Skills in other functional areas (e.g., speech and language, occupational therapy) are assessed as well, in order to ensure that the child's functioning is at a level where he or she can access educational opportunities in the least restrictive manner. When the child enters high school, then planning for vocational success should also be a part of planning efforts (Individuals with Disabilities Education Act, 2004).

Section 504 Plans. Section 504 Plans (from Section 504 of the Rehabilitation Act of 1973; http://www2.ed.gov/about/offices/list/ocr/504faq.html; Conderman & Katsiyannis, 1995) apply for children with special medical conditions or mental health care needs who do not necessarily quality for an IEP (Osborne & Russo, 2014). A section 504 plan is a written plan for children with "other health impairments"that provides guidelines for meeting the children's needs to promote their achievement at school (Madaus & Shaw, 2004). Specifically, a child who has a mental or physical impairment is eligible for services if the school receives any type of federal funding (Osborne & Russo, 2014). A physical or mental impairment is defined as a condition that limits an individual's ability to engage in daily activities. A Section 504 plan would be enforced by the Office of Civil Rights. A section 504 plan is similar to an Individual Education Plan, but may not have as much detail. School officials do not have to grant all requests for accommodations written in a 504 plan (Osborne & Russo, 2014). Similar to an Individual Education Plan, periodic re-evaluation of the child's functioning is recommended.

Accommodation plans assist individual children in attaining their educational goals and needs. A team should review the student's needs, determine appropriate educational planning, and review the plan periodically. Section 504 plans are broad and beneficial in that they can address a multitude of the child's needs. For instance, compensatory planning can be recorded in a Section 504 Plan, such as assisting a child to acquire a second set of textbooks, providing assistance getting to classes or moving through the school building, or ensuring that tests are read orally. Items on a Section 504 can be at the policy level, allowing a child more times to be "tardy" or flexibility in meeting physical education requirements. These plans can address medication administration and other health needs (e.g., needing special meal plans). Recent legislation and attention has highlighted the importance of implementing these plans in a timely fashion, such that Section 504 Plans can become a protective factor—outlining needs for success for children with medical conditions and mental health problems in schools (Conderman & Katsiyannis, 1995; Kim & Samples, 2013).

Spiel, Evans, and Langberg (2014) evaluated the content of IEPs and Section 504 plans for 97 youth (6th through 8th grade) with Attention-Deficit/Hyperactivity Disorder to determine if the services offered were research based and were consistent with evidence-based interventions. The plans were coded for types of services provided in IEPs and 504 plans and chi-square analyses were used to examine the frequency of different types of services for different special health care needs. Findings indicated that although problematic behaviors were identified in the plans, there were not always goals for addressing the behavior. Students with IEPs were likely to receive more intensive intervention services. Only 18 % of the services listed on the plans were considered "research-based" or developed from evidence-based literature. Consequently, many of the services being used for students also had very little evidence-based research supporting their effectiveness. For example, behavior modification has a long history of evidence, and the researchers found that only about 25 % of the IEPs and a little over 5 % of the Section 504 plans listed behavior modification as service. Plans to support studying were often mentioned on plans and taking breaks during tests was mentioned, and the authors pointed out that research is lacking to support the effectiveness of these interventions. Finally, they concluded that the effectiveness of services for the children was not evaluated very often. This is problematic, given that effective services boost performance and academic competence.

Individualized Health Care Plans. An individualized health care plan is a written care plan that is on file at the school perhaps with the teacher or school nurse. They can use the steps in the plan, which outline the child's health care needs, to help the child complete classwork and manage his or her chronic illness in the school setting. Kim and Samples (2013) discussed the importance of implementing health care plans and moving to Section 504 Plans as needed for children with chronic illnesses. They argued that Individual Healthcare Plans (IHPs) for students are not a mechanism to circumvent the obligations of providing alternative ways to reach a free and appropriate education through a Section 504 Plan when a child has a chronic medical condition. One criticism of IHPs was that they are not required to be developed by individuals knowledgeable about the student or knowledgeable about the components of a Section 504 Plan. Typically, one individual, a school nurse, implements these plans. A Section 504 Plan may be advantageous because evaluation of student abilities is conducted by a team. In addition, these authors suggested that a Section 504 Plan process considers all aspects of a child's functioning, rather than just health care needs, making it a more "holistic" approach. The emphasis on academic needs that could be considered in a Section 504 plan was considered advantageous for the child, and the authors mentioned that if academic needs were significant, then an IEP should be considered. They presented several cases where children with health care needs had insufficient school plans and were in need of Section 504 Plans, suggesting that advocating for school accommodations to improve the school functioning of children with special health care needs is still an area where advocacy and persistence may be fruitful, in terms of ensuring that the academic needs of these children are met.

The diabetes workgroup for the School, Adolescent and Reproductive Group, Division of Community Health Promotion, of the Florida Health Department (Diabetes Guidelines Workgroup (January, 2015) developed information for IHPs for children with diabetes. Their document entitled, "Guidelines for the Care and Delegation of Care for Students with Diabetes in Florida Schools," was very thorough and offered detailed information on roles for school personnel, a sample health care plan for children, and guidelines about care of diabetes in the school setting (http://sss.usf.edu/resources/format/pdf/diabetes-guidelines-for-the-care--delegation-of-care-for-students-with-diabetes-in-florida-schools.pdf, accessed June 8, 2015). The working group had developed a flowchart with guidance for actions during a hypoglycemic episode. Finally, there was advice for those leading after-school activities and for bus drivers. This document would be an example of a guide for school staff developing individual health plans for a child with diabetes at school. In addition, the general areas covered in this plan (roles for school staff, emergency planning, daily care, specialized care) are good areas to cover in IHPs across a variety of health and mental health conditions.

Implementation of School Plans. Few studies have assessed implementation of IEPs and Section 504 Plans. Noell and Gansle (2006) noted that examination of how the plan is implemented and the success of each step of a special health care plan in schools are infrequently documented. In addition, the person or persons implementing the interventions for the plans rarely review data on the children's progress (Noell et al., 2005). Recording behavioral data, such as the frequency of change in key behaviors, and presenting data in table formats can summarize the child's progress on key goals. Moreover, data from teacher interviews and from child performance on standardized testing can provide other data to inform decisions. Because data is rarely available, there is a gap between learning from the plan and sharing information with the teacher and others "on the ground" implementing the activities outlined in health care plans. A goal is to share information on progress and implementation of each intervention with teachers and specialists working with the children, so that the plan can be better developed and modified to meet children's needs.

Consultation of and Meeting with Teachers. Teachers are supporting more children with special health care needs in their classrooms. This can be difficult as they lack knowledge and training to adequately meet these children's needs (Hinton & Kirk, 2015). An untapped area for health education is to work with teachers, either in one-on-one sessions, workshops, or other consultation models to educate them about how to care for children with special health care needs. Health professionals can also play a role in being a support person that improves communication between the family, nurse, and teacher. This will be another tool to improve teacher knowledge of interventions needed to support youth (Hinton & Kirk, 2015). It also may be beneficial to ensure that written health care plans reach teachers or that teachers receive a personalized version of the child's health care plan that outlines the teacher's responsibilities in optimizing the child's educational experience. Teachers' perspectives may go unheard in developing and implementing special health care plans in the schools. Thus, involving them in the design and implementation of IEPs and health care plans can facilitate the child's development as well as teacher self-efficacy for implementing goals on the child's individual plan.

Lee-Tarver (2006) surveyed over 100 teachers in Alabama and Georgia about their opinions of Individual Education Programs. Over 50 % of the teachers reported that IEPs assisted with instruction. Surprisingly, a sizable minority (over 20 %) did not feel that the written guidelines provided an educational curriculum for a child.

"Forty-percent of teachers reported that they were better teachers because they have an IEP to guide their instructional planning and 12.2 % strongly agreed that they were better teachers by having IEPs as a guide for planning" (p. 276).

Interestingly, over 20 % of the teachers indicated that the time spent in developing IEPs did not justify their worth. Approximately 20 % of the teachers reported that the information shared at IEP meetings did not help them develop goals and objectives for children. Thus, a sizable minority were not as positive about the use of IEPs to guide their classroom planning for a child with special needs. Lee-Tarver (2006) suggested teacher training to improve knowledge about the purpose and uses of an IEP. It also may be likely that consultation for IEPs for children with special health needs may be beneficial to enable teachers to address IEP goals and the needs of children that may emerge as the teacher implements IEP goals.

One key role for health professionals is to network with teachers in order to gather their opinions on ideas for intervention for children with special needs in their classrooms. Another area is to ascertain their perceptions about the extent to which they feel that they can successfully implement interventions developed by special education teams. Health educators also can be key players in collecting data to confirm the success of the child in meeting goals outlined on IEPs and in other types of school plans. It is recommended that a health professional on the child's school team be identified as the contact for networking between home and the classroom. The health educator or school counselor may be in an optimal position to fill this role. In this consulting role, it would be possible to provide ongoing support for teachers through education to help them support children with special needs in their classrooms.

Case Study

Abbigail or "Abby" is a 9-year-old girl who has pain related to having Juvenile Idiopathic Arthritis (JIA). She resides at home with her mother, father, and 4-year-old brother. She has some good friends in her neighborhood and at school. Her grades are good; she makes mostly "A's" and "B's" at school. She is not experiencing significant anxiety or depression. She does not have any problems following directions. The arthritis she experiences causes pain in her hands and elbows. She takes aspirin when her arthritis flares up and she holds hot wax to help her hands feel better when she has an arthritis flare (a painful episode related to her JIA). She soaks her elbows in warm water when they feel "bad." She goes to physical therapy regularly to help her mobility in her hands and elbows.

Abby often has to miss school when she has flare-ups of her pain, especially when the weather changes in the spring and fall. She has trouble carrying her heavy textbooks home to complete her homework. The nurse on Abby's medical team is working with her teacher to develop an educational plan at school. After several conversations, they have decided on a plan of care card that will help her teacher remember what to do when Abby experiences a pain flare. The first part of the plan, however, involves networking with Abby's principal to help her obtain a second set of textbooks to keep at home. It will relieve her to have extra books at home so that she does not have to carry her books when having a pain flare up.

After some telephone calls the nurse arranges a meeting with the principal, Abby's mother, the school psychologist, and Abby's teacher. During their meeting, the principal agrees that Abby can have an extra set of textbooks at home. The principal also contacts the nurse during the meeting and she comes down to attend the meeting and have Abby's mother fill out paperwork so that there is aspirin available in the nurse's office to provide to Abby should her pain become high during the school day. Abby's teacher mentions that she will develop an outline of assignments and reading that Abby can review on the days she has to miss school because of pain. Abby's mother will stop by to pick up packets of missed work at the front office. Abby's teacher and mother share emails, so that they can communicate about Abby's medical condition and school progress. A release of information form is filled out at the meeting, so that the school has a record that it is acceptable to release information to Abby's medical team, via quarterly contacts with the school nurse. The primary contact for the medical team will be the nurse that Abby works with most frequently when she attends clinic visits with the Rheumatology team at a nearby children's hospital. The nurse at the hospital is the designated team member for school contacts and she keeps up with schools on a quarterly basis over the course of the school year.

The school psychologist, who also attended the meeting, agreed with the team that her services were not needed at this time. The school psychologist did mention that if she was needed she could explain Abby's medical condition to her class, to ensure her peers understood how her arthritis impacted her at school. Abby's mother was satisfied that the current level of educational planning would meet Abby's needs and she felt that the care card reminding the teacher to add information for home when Abby missed class and send her to the nurse for pain medications was adequate planning for now. The team agreed that Abby is doing well and there is not a need for a Section 504 plan, but that they will reconnect at the end of the school year to determine if a Section 504 plan is needed for next year.

Summary

In this chapter, a broad definition of the role of a health educator was proposed. In the second section of this introductory chapter, information on educational planning to improve academic and psychosocial functioning of children with special health care and mental health care needs was introduced. Information on Section 504 plans and Individual Education Programs was presented. In the case study, a brief presentation of a case of a child with Juvenile Idiopathic Arthritis was reviewed. This case was not very severe in nature, in terms of impact on the child and her school performance. Therefore, an informal care plan was developed with a team of professionals from the child's school, the nurse from the child's medical team, and her mother. The team might have been even more informed of a "best blueprint for care" if they had included Abby herself in the planning process. Nonetheless, the case study provided an example of an initial step in care planning to assist a child with complications due to her chronic illness in the school setting. The communication and planning served to smooth the way for Abby to have a relatively stress-free school experience.

Exercises/Review Questions

1. Provide a definition of a Section 504 Plan and an Individual Education Program. In your opinion, what is the key difference between the two?
2. What is your personal definition of a health educator? Compare and contrast the definition of a health educator that is provided in this chapter with your own definition. What aspects are the same and which ones differ?
3. How would you follow Abby's progress at school and evaluate whether a more formal health care plan is needed?
4. What is your orientation, as a health educator, for working with children with special health care and mental health care needs?
5. What types of community and school connections do you believe are critical for promoting the social development of children with health care needs? Would these connections be the same or different for children with mental health problems? If the connections would differ, what would be critical actions and connections to promote the social development of children with mental health problems, in your opinion?

Key Concepts

Functional Analysis of Behavior
Health Educator
Section 504 Plan
Individualized Education Program (IEP)
Individualized Health Care Plan (IHP)

References

Baker, D. L., Hebbeler, K., Davis-Alldritt, L., Anderson, L. S., & Knauer, H. (2015). School health services for children with special health care needs in California. *The Journal of School Nursing, 31*(5), 318–25. doi:10.1177/1059840515578753.

Boulet, S. L., Boyle, C. A., & Schieve, L. A. (2009). Health care use and health and functional impact of developmental disabilities among U.S. children, 1997–2005. *Adolescent Medicine, 163*(1), 19–26.

Conderman, G., & Katsiyannis, A. (1995). Section 504 Accommodation Plans. *Intervention in School and Clinic, 31*(1), 42.

Council on Children with Disabilities. (2007). Provision of educationally related services for children and adolescents with chronic diseases and disabling conditions. *Pediatrics, 119*(6), 1218–1223. doi:10.1542/peds2007-0885.

Diabetes Guidelines Workgroup (January, 2015). *Guidelines for the care and delegation of care for students with diabetes in Florida schools*. For the School, Adolescent and Reproductive Health Section, Division of Community Health Promotion, Florida Department of Health. Retrieved June 8, 2015, from http://sss.usf.edu/resources/format/pdf/diabetes-guidelines-for-the-care--delegation-of-care-for-students-with-diabetes-in-florida-schools.pdf.

Evans, S. W., Sapia, J. L., Axelrod-Lowie, J., & Glomb, N. K. (2002). Practical issues in school mental health: Referral procedures, negotiating special education, and confidentiality. In H. S. Ghuman, M. D. Weist, & R. M. Sarles (Eds.), *Providing mental health services to youth where they are: School and community-based approaches* (pp. 75–94). New York, NY: Routledge.

Forrest, C. B., Bevans, K. B., Riley, A. W., Crespo, R., & Louis, T. A. (2011). School outcomes of children with special health care needs. *Pediatrics, 128*, 303–312.

Halfon, N., Houtrow, A., Larson, K., & Newacheck, P. W. (2012). The changing landscape of disability in childhood. *Future of Children, 22*(1), 13–42.

Hinton, D., & Kirk, S. (2015). Teachers' perspectives of supporting pupils with long-term health conditions in mainstream schools: a narrative review of the literature. *Health and Social Care in the Community, 23*(2), 107–120.

Houtrow, A. J., Larson, K., Olson, L. M., Newacheck, P. W., & Halfon, N. (2014). Changing trends of childhood disability, 2001–2011. *Pediatrics, 134*(3), 530–538.

Individuals With Disabilities Education Act, 20 U.S.C. § 1400 (2004).

Kim, D., & Samples, E. (2013). Comparing Individual Healthcare Plans and Section 504 Plans: School districts' obligation to determine eligibility for students with health related conditions. *Urban Lawyer, 45*(1), 263–279.

Lee-Tarver, A. (2006). Are individualized education plans a good thing? A survey of teachers' perceptions of the utility of IEPs in regular education settings. *Journal of Instructional Psychology, 33*(4), 263–272.

Madaus, J. W., & Shaw, S. F. (2004). Section 504: Differences in the regulations for secondary and post-secondary education. *Intervention in School and Clinic, 40*(2), 81–87.

Mills, C. L., & Cunningham, D. L. (2014). Building bridges: The role of expanded school mental health in supporting students with emotional and behavioral difficulties in the least restrictive environment. In M. D. Weist, N. A. Lever, C. P. Bradshaw, & J. S. Owens (Eds.), *Handbook of school mental health: Issues in clinical child psychology: research, training and policy* (2nd ed., pp. 87–98). New York, NY: Springer. doi:10.1007/978-1-4614-7624-5_7.

Nelson, M. R., Alexander, M. A., & Molnar, G. E. (2015). History and examination. In M. A. Alexander, D. J. Mathews, & K. P. Murphy (Eds.), *Pediatric rehabilitation* (Principles and practice 5th ed., pp. 1–11). New York, NY: Demos Medical Publishing.

Noell, G. H., & Gansle, K. A. (2006). Assuring the form has substance: Treatment plan implementation as the foundation of assessing response to intervention. *Assessment for Effective Intervention, 32*, 32–39.

Noell, G. H., Witt, J. C., Slider, N. J., Connell, J. E., Gatti, S. L., Williams, K. L., et al. (2005). Treatment implementation following behavioral consultation in schools: A comparison of three follow-up strategies. *School Psychology Review, 34*, 87–106.

O'Connor, M., Howell-Meurs, S., Kvalsvig, A., & Goldfeld, S. (2014). Understanding the impact of special health care needs on early school functioning: a conceptual model. *Child: Care, Health and Development, 41*(1), 15–22.

Osborne, A. G., Jr., & Russo, C. J. (2014). *Special education and the law: A guide for practitioners* (3rd ed.). Thousand Oaks, CA: Corwin Press.

Spiel, C. F., Evans, S. W., & Langberg, J. M. (2014). Evaluating the content of individualized education programs and 504 plans of young adolescents with Attention Deficit/Hyperactivity Disorder. *School Psychology Quarterly, 29*(4), 452–468.

Chapter 2
Asthma

Diagnosis

Asthma or reactive airways disease is one of the most common chronic illnesses in children (Akinbami, Moorman, Garbe, & Sondik, 2009; Centers for Disease Control [CDC], 2011). This illness is diagnosed when children suffer from episodic wheezing, shortness of breath, chest tightness, and coughing (Bousquet et al., 2010; National Institutes of Health, Heart, Lung, and Blood Institute, 2014). It is defined as an airway inflammation, narrowing, or obstruction that is either reversible or partially reversible with treatment. Airways can be obstructed or narrowed due to an accumulation of mucous. The clinical presentation of asthma involves a decrease in "exhaled" air flow. The clinical presentation also can involve edema (swelling) of the bronchial walls and subsequent contraction of the smooth muscles around the airways. This can cause a feeling of tightness, almost like rubber bands "constricting" or "pulling tight" with accompanying chest pain or tightness. This can feel very uncomfortable, making it difficult to breathe. When doctors are assessing children for asthma, they are examining reports of wheezing, chest tightness, reports of shortness of breath, and coughing. They assess air flow using spirometry (a device children blow through and nurses/doctors assess exhaled breaths). Children with asthma may also experience nighttime awakenings due to difficulty breathing or exacerbations of daytime symptoms. Treatment often involves administration of oral or systemic corticosteroids.

Symptoms of asthma may be diagnosed at any time during childhood. The diagnosis is most often made during the first 4 years of a child's life. Asthma is most common in childhood and then it is likely to decline in adolescence. In general, females are more likely than males to be diagnosed with asthma (American Academy of Allergy, Asthma, and Immunology, 2014; CDC, 2011). Asthma is a difficult disease to diagnose and, at present, cannot be cured (National Institutes of

© Springer International Publishing Switzerland 2016
L. Nabors, *Medical and Mental Health During Childhood*, Springer
Series on Child and Family Studies, DOI 10.1007/978-3-319-31117-3_2

Health, National Heart, Lung, and Blood Institute, 2007). However, symptoms of asthma can be effectively managed through medication and by reducing exposure to environmental triggers and allergens (American Academy of Allergy, Asthma, and Immunology, 2014; National Institutes of Health, National Heart, Lung, & Blood Institute, 2007).

Prevalence

Over 8 % of the individuals in the United States have asthma, and the prevalence of this disease is higher among children than adults (Akinbami et al., 2012). Asthma is a common illness for children, occurring in 40 per 1000 children. Asthma affects about 9.5–10 % of school-age children in the United States (Akinbami et al., 2012; American Academy of Allergy, Asthma, and Immunology, 2014; CDC, 2014). Asthma is more common in black, American Indian, and Alaskan native groups than for whites. Asthma rates were lower in groups of Asian descent (Akinbami et al., 2012). The prevalence of asthma has been increasing and this chronic illness also may be increasing for youth residing in poverty, especially those residing in poverty in areas where environmental risk factors, such as pollution, are high (Akinbami et al., 2012; Gergen & Togias, 2015; Wilson et al., 2015).

Genetic and Environmental Determinants. There is a genetic component to this disease, but the environment plays a large part in the onset and maintenance of symptoms. In terms of genetic influence, multiple genes play a role in determining asthma. In addition, prenatal exposure to different stimuli has been associated with the development of asthma in children. Two studies demonstrating this idea come from Project Viva, a longitudinal study (study conducted over time with measurements as the children age) to determine the impact of prenatal nutrition on child health. Specifically, Project Viva examined the relationship between food intake during pregnancy and health indicators during infancy and asthma during childhood (Bunyavanich et al., 2014; see https://www.hms.harvard.edu/viva/project-viva-publications.html). In a study examining links between food allergens and allergies and asthma during pregnancy, Bunyavanich et al. (2014) discovered that higher milk intake during the first trimester of a pregnancy was associated with lower levels of allergic rhinitis and asthma in childhood. Similarly, Bunyavanich et al. found that higher intake of wheat and peanuts during pregnancy was related to lower levels of allergic rhinitis and asthma in children. Other variables, such as medication use, may impact child propensity toward asthma. Sordillo et al. (2015) examined the relationship between acetaminophen use and asthma in 1,490 mother–child dyads from Project Viva. Study findings did indicate a positive relationship between prenatal acetaminophen use and childhood asthma. However, the authors also emphasized the further study of number of respiratory tract infections during infancy is important as this factor could account for increased risk for asthma in the childhood years.

Impact on Children

Asthma is often considered a chronic illness with more "mild" severity levels and consequences. However, asthma attacks can be life threatening. Moreover, there is a significant subgroup of individuals with asthma with uncontrolled or very poorly controlled asthma, such that their symptoms are considered severe (Bousquet et al., 2010). If asthma symptoms are exacerbated, emergency room visits can become commonplace for youngsters. When symptoms of asthma are poorly managed, children can have serious attacks that lead to use of the emergency room or increased medical visits, which can be very expensive (Barnett & Nurmagambetov, 2011; McPherson & Redsell, 2009). Use of the emergency room may be more common for youth with severe asthma. In addition, these youth may be more likely to react negatively to their asthma medications and have poor lung function (e.g., loss of elasticity in lungs; Bousquet et al., 2010). However, severity levels change over time and a child can move from more severe to mild or moderate symptoms. Asthma remains difficult to diagnose and at present cannot be cured (National Institutes of Health, National Heart, Lung, & Blood Institute, 2007).

Assessment of Asthma. Current guidelines for asthma management (National Institutes of Health, National Heart, Lung, & Blood Institute, 2007; Wilson et al., 2015) recommend assessment of patient (in the case of children, child and parent) knowledge about disease management so that appropriate health education can be provided. Part of this knowledge involves understanding of factors, such as allergens and stress, which can trigger an asthma attack, as well as knowledge about the need to use an inhaler regularly. Children need to know how to use an inhaler, by expelling a breath, taking in a full breath with a puff from the inhaler, and closing their mouths around the tube for the inhaler. Children should then hold their breath for a few seconds and then expel it. Information about chest tightness and wheezing also should be familiar to children and parents because these symptoms can signal an asthma attack. These types of questions should be assessed (and be key items on questionnaires) when working with children with asthma and their parents or caregivers.

Researchers working with evaluation data from the Head-off Environmental Asthma in Louisianna (Heal) Project (http://heal.niehs.nih.gov/) have analyzed data for asthma risk using the CARAT or Child Asthma Risk Assessment Tool (Wilson et al., 2015). The CARAT is available at http://carat.asthmarisk.org/ (accessed July 7, 2015). Development of this tool was sponsored by the Agency for Healthcare Research and Quality (AHRQ). There are many helpful pieces of information at the aforementioned website, such as information that will help health educators explain asthma to children and parents and information on the development and utility of the Child Asthma Risk Assessment Tool or CARAT. The CARAT is a survey that comprises 36 items examining asthma status as well as triggers or risk factors for asthma management including exposure to smoke, environmental risk factors (e.g., humidifier in child's room, mildew in the home), medication adherence, child well-being, and attitudes toward asthma. The CARAT may be a practical tool for health educators to determine if education is needed and to determine baseline information about child and caregiver well-being.

When examining information for children whose caregivers completed the CARAT ($n = 155$), Wilson et al. (2015) found that 46 % of the children were at high risk when considering medication administration. A third of the children were at risk in terms of child well-being and a similar number of parents were at risk for relatively poor well-being. Medical care and exposure to allergens were relatively lower "risk areas." The children with asthma were typically over 5 years of age and were receiving Medicaid and had "persistent" asthma symptoms. Wilson et al. highlighted the importance of education and control of environmental triggers for asthma attacks with children. They also highlighted the importance of improving caregiver and child feelings of self-efficacy for adherence and disease management. Wilson et al. (2015) discussed the importance of working with parents to change any negative beliefs they might have about management of their child's asthma. Improving parent knowledge about asthma management may help them reduce negative beliefs, which in turn could improve their abilities to coach their child and help their child with improved asthma management. Wilson et al. suggested that parents remain active in supervising their child's asthma management, in order to improve adherence to medical recommendations.

Disease Management. For children to maintain control of their asthma symptoms and reduce risk of asthma flare-ups and attacks, ongoing monitoring of disease management is important. The Monitoring Asthma in Children statement was developed from review of the literature and input from 22 clinical and research experts in children's asthma (Pijnenburg et al., 2015). A task force was formed to develop an expert statement. First, it was suggested that physicians or pediatricians and parents and children regularly monitor children's symptoms. Parents and children should record peak expiratory flow (peak flow), which is typically recorded using a peak expiratory flow monitor. Children blow into one end of the device and there is a scale at the other end. The child's peak flow (assessment of breathing ability) is assessed compared to normal rates of others in the same height and weight range. Previous assessment of peak flow data also can be reviewed. Records of peak flow can be brought to the physician's office.

The child's physician is also clinically assessing change in symptoms, including times when asthma flares (symptoms) increase, adherence to the medical regimen (parent and child following medical recommendations), inhaler technique, control of asthma triggers (stimuli that trigger asthma symptoms), use of asthma care plans, and child height and weight. Poorly controlled asthma is defined as three to four indicators of problems, which can include symptoms for more than two times per week, nighttime awakening due to asthma, reliever medication use more than two times a week, and activity limitations due to asthma (Pijnenburg et al., 2015). Physicians should also be examining bronchial responsiveness and markers of lung inflammation as needed. A thorough review of medical management is beyond the scope of this introductory chapter. Those interested in learning details of medical management could consult local medical experts specializing in the treatment of asthma or experts at local children's hospitals. Information in this section of the chapter focuses on typical practice, rather than the management of severe asthma. It is noteworthy that management of severe asthma is complex and involves consideration of a myriad of factors (see Guilbert, Bacharier, & Fitzpatrick, 2014 for a review of management of severe asthma in children).

Use of Inhalers. One typical medication for children with asthma is the delivery of steroid or other asthma medications (e.g., bronchodilators used for quick relief of symptoms) through an inhaler. Many children do use inhalers to administer asthma medication and there is risk that they will not use the inhaler appropriately. Closing one's mouth over the inhaler when administering medication and insuring that the inhaler is primed are two important steps in inhaler use. It is noteworthy that inhalers are primed differently and parents should consult the directions (often inhalers are primed before the first use and if they have not been used, by shaking them and maybe by pumping the inhaler one time). Making sure that the child exhales prior to administration of medication is also important. This author would recommend several steps including: (1) remove the cap, (2) prime the inhaler, (3) blow out the air in your lungs, (4) put your mouth around the inhaler and administer the puff or puffs the doctor recommended, and (5) hold the puff in your lungs for a few seconds before exhaling. These instructions help with using a metered dose inhaler (the most common type of inhaler). Information on other types of inhalers is available at http://www.aaaai.org/conditions-and-treatments/conditions-dictionary/asthma-inhalers.aspx (accessed July 7, 2015).

Detailed recommendations on administration of asthma medications using an inhaler are available at http://www.aaaai.org/conditions-and-treatments/library/at-a-glance/inhaled-asthma-medications.aspx. These guidelines are provided by the American Academy of Allergy, Asthma and Immunology. This national group of experts has provided excellent information on use of inhalers, medications, and asthma treatment. There are many sources for education of asthma medications and use of inhalers. For example, other resources are available from the American Academy of Pediatrics, Section on Allergy and Immunology (example, guidelines for Asthma by this section are available at: http://www2.aap.org/sections/allergy/guidelines.cfm). The reader of this chapter is encouraged to ask medical experts and search websites reviewed by national experts to learn more about asthma medications and administration of these medications.

Triggers for Asthma Symptoms. The environmental causes of asthma, such as poor environmental conditions and allergies, serve as triggers for asthma symptoms to flare and a child to have an asthma attack. Emotions can trigger an attack as well. In fact, stress, anxiety, and being emotionally reactive are possible causes of asthma attacks. Children with asthma are at increased risk of having new asthma attacks directly after and even weeks after experiencing stressful life events (Sandberg, Jarvenpaa, Penttinen, Paton, & McCann, 2004). Table 2.1 presents a listing of "asthma triggers" developed from the author's experience working with children who have asthma and from research (e.g., Bousquet et al., 2010; Chen, Bloomberg, Fisher, & Strunk, 2003; Wilson et al., 2015). Children with asthma often have airways that are hyper-responsive or very sensitive to stimulation from their asthma triggers (e.g., exercise, exposure to environmental irritants). Consequently, children and their parents or caregivers need to learn to use medications as directed and avoid triggers when their asthma symptoms appear to be worsening.

Table 2.1 Triggers or factors related to asthma symptom exacerbation

1. Inhaler misuse—the child can use the inhaler inappropriately. This can occur when the child does not close his or her mouth over the inhaler. To use the inhaler the child should expel a breath, place the inhaler in his or her mouth around the inhaler to prevent medication escaping, and release the intended dosage or "puff"

2. Not taking medications as prescribed—this is a lack of adherence to the medication regimen. Many parents can under-dose their children as they may be concerned that the medicine changes their child's behavior (e.g., "it makes my child hyper")

3. Inadequate treatment/inadequate disease control by doctors—many pediatricians and asthma specialists recommend aggressive treatment of asthma symptoms so as to prevent asthma flare-ups (e.g., severe asthma attacks)

4. Exposure to environmental irritants—strong cleaners, dust, allergens, mold

5. Passive smoking—exposure to second-hand smoke

6. Viral respiratory tract infections, colds, sinusitis

7. Psychological and emotional stress

8. Residing in low-income areas with high pollution and environmental irritants

As shown in Table 2.1, dust and mold in older homes, such as those in inner city or urban areas, can cause symptoms of asthma or increase symptoms in children who have asthma. Other environmental conditions can impact symptoms of asthma and these include: having viral infections or pneumonia that damage the lungs or having allergies. Exposure to cigarette smoking can also cause symptoms. Second-hand smoke can cause an exacerbation of symptoms and adults should attempt to be careful to smoke outside the home if they have a child with asthma, if they continue smoking. Exposure to allergens, such as pet dander, can also trigger an attack.

Adherence to Medical Regimens. Adherence to the doctor's recommendations or following the doctor or medical professional's recommendations for asthma management can be a significant concern for children with asthma. Not following medical recommendations, particularly administration of oral steroids, may be directly related to serious asthma flare-ups resulting in over-use of emergency rooms. Family, particularly parental support, may be needed to ensure that the child remains "on track" in terms of following medical recommendations. The health professional can be very helpful in supporting parent supervision of and leadership in adherence efforts. Before providing recommendations to improve adherence it may be advisable to assess how parents are managing the child's asthma. If children and parents manage the child's asthma using a team approach, then directing questions to both parent and child may be an appropriate way to gather information. Table 2.2 provides key questions for understanding how well parents are managing their child's asthma and trouble-shooting various "asthma triggers."

Table 2.2 presents questions and tips to improve asthma management—many of the ideas presented in Table 2.2 are key areas to following what doctors recommend in terms of adherence to recommendations for care of asthma.

Table 2.2 Questions to determine adherence and roles for health educators

Question	Adherence or asthma management tip
Are you keeping a written record of peak flow measurements?	Record your child's peak flow measurements. With this record you will be able to determine when additional or rescue medication is needed
Are you recording information about asthma triggers—that can signal an attack or escalate symptoms?	Keep a list of your child's asthma triggers. Then, ask your child's medical team or read current literature and learn ways to eliminate or reduce the impact of asthma triggers, such as dust and exercise
How are you doing in terms of filling prescriptions on time?	Make sure that your child's most current prescriptions are filled and are up-to-date
Are you administering the recommended dose of oral steroids and other medications?	Talk to your child's doctor about his or her recommended dose and why it is important to use the full dose and administer it regularly. If children are not using the full dose, they might be more prone to asthma attacks and then face additional emergent care visits
How are you asthma proofing the indoor environment? (at home and at school?)	Assist the parent on brainstorming about use of cleaning products, mattress covers, HEPA filters, and other environmental changes that can help the child. Stress the need to maintain environmental surveillance to manage triggers. At school, have the child bring wipes to school (to clean/sanitize areas). Educate teachers about asthma management needs of each child using a written care plan

Asking questions about administration of medications are important steps in learning if parents need to be more effective in following medical recommendations. In addition, having a trigger-free environment is critical. Some suggestions for a trigger-free environment include: keeping areas clean and free of dust, reducing exposure to second-hand smoke, not having pets, and using air filters. If there is a pet in the home, remind parents that regular baths (e.g., weekly and as needed during allergy seasons) are important and, if possible, keep pets outside the bedroom. Other helpful recommendations for the home setting include: reducing humidity levels, washing bedding regularly, and encasing pillows and mattresses in plastic. It may be beneficial for parents to keep a notebook or chart detailing their care of the child and their efforts to control or reduce the impact of asthma triggers. Parents can show these records to the child's doctor at appointments so that the doctor can understand what happens with medical management between appointments. This may lead to better recommendations from the doctor.

Psychosocial and Emotional Functioning

Children who have asthma may experience emotional problems, most commonly depression or anxiety (DuPlessis-Erickson, Spett, Stoltzfu-Mullett, Jensen, & Bisson-Belseth, 2006; García-Walker, 2012). They may feel "different" from their peers because they have an illness, have to administer medication, or have to miss school for doctors' appointments related to their asthma. Some children with asthma may experience low self-esteem related to feeling isolated and different from peers. In the long run, frequent problems with asthma management can lead to feelings of poor quality of life for children with this disease (DuPlessis-Erickson et al., 2006; Mosnaim et al., 2013; Stewart et al., 2012). Children with asthma may feel conspicuous at school or in other public settings where they have to administer their inhalers. Inhalers typically allow children to administer steroid medications immediately. Guilbert et al. (2014) reported that experiencing depression and anxiety are markers for increased emergency room visits in children with asthma. If a child has frequent emergent care visits and presents with anxiety and depression, then referral for counseling may be indicated.

It is important to rule out side effects of medications when considering the child's school functioning, mood, and academic performance. For example, steroid medications can make children appear very active, and in extreme cases it may look like the child is experiencing very active behaviors akin to being hyperactive. The medications can negatively affect memory and attention, which can be problematic in the classroom. As mentioned, children who have poor control of their symptoms at night may not get enough sleep and may be tired during the school day. Thus, tiredness could negatively influence attention, recall, and concentration in the classroom. The health specialist needs to assess the reasons for a child's change in mood and then provide appropriate education about illness management. In most cases, it is advisable to maintain a strong relationship with the child's doctor and have a release of information to talk with the doctor. A release of information is a written statement, signed by the child's legal guardian, which then permits health care providers to converse about the child's medical condition and care. It is recommended that health educators and counselors frequently contact the medical professional so that he or she is aware of how the child and parent(s) are managing triggers for asthma attacks and get an update about the child's general functioning.

Interventions for Children with Asthma and Their Caregivers

Educational interventions can be effective in changing behavior, especially in the short-term. Horn et al. (2014) conducted an educational intervention to improve parents' sense of connectedness with primary care physicians and their communication with them. Horn et al.'s study was a randomized controlled trial recruiting 150 parents of children (aged 1–12 years) who were randomly assigned to receive an educational intervention ($n=77$) versus receiving care as usual ($n=73$). Parents resided in an urban area and the majority of study participants were African American. Over 90 % of the children had persistent asthma, and many were using the emergency room on a frequent basis. Parents in the intervention group participated in the Parent Empowerment for Asthma Care (PEPAC) Program where they received education on sharing information about and clarifying information about their child's asthma plan with their child's primary care physician. At 2 months post-intervention parents receiving the training (delivered by research assistants) reported increased identification with their child's primary care physician and there were reduced visits to the emergency room. The gains were not evident at a later assessment (6 months later). This could have occurred because the dose of the intervention or strength of the intervention was not sufficient to cause long-term change. It may be that parents need reminders and frequent visits to maintain a sharing and connected relationship with their child's primary care physician. Nonetheless, this study was encouraging as it provided evidence that an educational program could have an impact on emergency room use, which may improve care in the long run, should the physician–parent relationship remain strengthened and communication channels remain open. More research is needed to examine the long-term impact of educational interventions and to determine the correct dose of the intervention for maintaining long-term changes in parent behavior.

Although we know that clinical interventions can improve emotional and behavioral functioning in children with asthma, less in known about positive parenting interventions and how they impact child functioning. Clarke, Calam, Morawska, and Sanders (2013) developed an intervention to improve child health-related quality of life. After reviewing the literature, these researchers noted that educational interventions were more common than behavioral ones. They selected the Triple P (Positive Parenting Program) to implement with parents of children who had asthma. This Triple P Program is an evidence-based program to improve parent self-efficacy for child-rearing and reduce behavioral and emotional problems in children (Sanders, 1999). For Clarke and her colleagues' study, parents of children between the ages of 2 through 8 years who had asthma were randomly assigned to an intervention versus a nonintervention group. When patients are randomly assigned to groups, they have an equal chance of being assigned to the intervention or to the control group. Parents received asthma tip sheets showing the links between positive behavior for children and asthma management. In addition, parents participated in the Triple P Program, learning many positive behavioral techniques for childhood behavior management and ideas to promote children's positive functioning. This intervention was innovative in that it was delivered online, using video clips.

Unfortunately, parents did not always review information provided on web pages (Clarke et al., 2013). Very few parents engaged in the study after review of the video clips in the first lesson. Thus, the impact of this intervention could not be fully examined due to low enrollment in the study. This study was presented in this chapter because it was well designed and has ideas that may be helpful to students who want to engage in future research with parents. However, the asthma information and the link between emotional problems in children and asthma management may not have been made clearly enough, via the internet, to involve parents in the training. Parent training during in-person sessions, where one can engage parents around their own personal issues with their child and the child's specific asthma management difficulties may be a "stronger" intervention for reaching parents. Finally, the Triple P Program was designed for prevention of behavioral and emotional problems. Use of the positive parenting techniques in the Triple P Program may be more meaningful for parents of a child with asthma when their child is experiencing emotional and behavioral difficulties which are impacting asthma management.

Horner and Brown (2014) evaluated the impact of a self-management intervention for elementary school-age children (7–12 years of age) with asthma and their caregivers. Children received the intervention at school and parents learned of about the intervention during a home visit. This intervention was delivered in a rural setting, and the authors mentioned that more research is needed in rural areas. Children participated in the intervention during their lunch periods, in 15-min sessions (3 days per week for 5 and one-half weeks). Children learned to correctly use their metered dose inhaler and self-efficacy for correct and consistent use of the inhaler was emphasized. Children learned problem-solving and coping skills around asthma management and they learned tips about management of asthma during and after school through group discussion. Content of lessons included learning about use of the inhaler, how to avoid asthma triggers, how to get help in different situations, how lungs work, and how to interpret scores on a peak flow meter. Eighty-one children and caregivers participated in the intervention and 72 were in a comparison group. Children in the comparison group received attention during lunch-time groups and they learned about problem-solving, but this information was not tailored to asthma management. Children in both groups showed improved health, quality of life, and reduced emergency room visits (Horner & Brown, 2014). Parents were told at the start of the study if their child was assigned to the intervention versus the comparison group, and perhaps this impacted study findings. It may also be the case that children in the comparison group were applying problem-solving skills to key issues related to their asthma management.

Cicutto, To, and Murphy (2013) examined the impact of a school-based intervention to educate children with asthma, their parents, and the school community (teachers, principals, school staff). Nurses lead intervention efforts for children in elementary school (grades 1–5, 1316 children who were in 130 schools). Children learned about asthma management by reviewing the Roaring Adventures of Puff Asthma Management Program (http://www.educationforasthma.com/; accessed August 2, 2015). Information from the Creating Asthma Friendly Schools Resource Kit (http://www.asthmainschools.com/) was also reviewed by nurses. Information on controlling asthma triggers and asthma management was reviewed with children, parents, and school staff. Control schools—where asthma education was not implemented—were included in this study. Children with asthma who participated in the intervention showed better "inhaler technique." Inhaler technique was assessed by providing points for removing the cap, priming the inhaler, exhaling, using the inhaler appropriately (placing mouth over inhaler without spaces while administering medicine), and holding one's breath. Findings indicated that urgent health care visits decreased for children with asthma in the intervention schools. School absences also reduced in the intervention relative to the control schools. Cicutto et al. (2013) concluded that results were positive, suggesting that broad-based educational efforts delivered by school nurses can be effective in improving asthma management in schools. Cicutto et al. mentioned that having insurance may not always ensure that children with asthma have access to the care that they need, such that school-based education and intervention efforts are a mechanism for improving health care and knowledge about asthma management for children, their families, and the broader school community.

Turcotte, Alker, Chaves, Gore, and Woskie (2014) conducted home assessments and provided a home-based intervention, focusing on education, cleaning, and controlling environmental triggers in the home, in an urban area. After the intervention, children's asthma symptoms were improved and costs—in terms of money spent on asthma care—decreased. Hence, "asthma-proofing" the environment at home may be a method for reducing costs and improving health outcomes for youth with asthma who reside in urban areas. Trouble-shooting and then improving the home environment is good for children with asthma irrespective of whether they reside in an inner city area, although such interventions may be especially helpful for children in urban areas. Others have described improving the home environment as consisting of parent and child education, frequent and thorough cleaning, pest management, and using high-efficiency particulate (HEPA) filters (Wright & Phipatanakul, 2014). Cleaning can reduce exposure to many household allergens, including but not limited to fecal matter from dust mites, saliva and secretions from cockroaches, mold and mildew, second-hand smoke, and dander from pets. Education is critical to learning these practices, but also is an opportunity to teach parents or caregivers that cleaning and other asthma-proofing practices need to be maintained on a long-term basis (Wright & Phipatanakul, 2014).

Roles for Health Educators and Mental Health Professionals

The health educator has a role in helping with adherence and monitoring of symptoms. There are many great sources for asthma education interventions. One of the many examples is material developed by the American Lung Association (http://www.lung.org/lung-disease/asthma/?referrer=https://www.google.com/; accessed August 2, 2015). Among materials at the American Lung Association are asthma fact sheets, asthma plans to use at school, and a myriad of resources for health educators and clinicians. This association has good resources for health professionals and parents. Health educators and counselors should review web-based resources in light of evidenced-based guidelines presented by pediatricians/physicians and information from peer-reviewed journal articles to learn about asthma management for children.

Helping the child feel comfortable and developing a care plan for school is another important role for health educators. Referral to trained mental health professionals, who specialize in the treatment of mood disorders or behavioral problems, may be necessary if the child is displaying significant problems with behavioral or emotional functioning that interfere with tasks of daily living, such as going to school, making friends, and functioning at home and during extracurricular activities. The health educator or counselor can also provide referral to asthma specialists when needed. Asthma proofing the child's environment and helping the child plan to avoid and control allergy triggers are other important roles for health educators. Parents or caregivers should be involved in the planning and educational process whenever possible, as a shared management approach or having the parent/caregiver check in and "supervise" medication administration and adherence to medical recommendations can be critical to positive disease management.

The health professional needs to assess how well the child perceives his or her respiratory symptoms as well as his or her knowledge of how to treat symptoms in order to design an educational plan. Understanding the child's perceptions indicates whether the child will be receptive to education and his or her abilities to understand written educational materials versus verbal instructions. Moreover, the practitioner can also gain an understanding of the child's willingness to implement treatment recommendations. It is important to ask about self-confidence or self-efficacy for being able to manage symptoms and do what the doctors recommend in terms of avoiding asthma triggers and using an inhaler. Health professionals can also help families make the home environment "better" for asthma patients. Improving the home environment may be especially important in the inner city, in high-poverty areas.

Case Study

Sashay is an 8-year-old girl attending an elementary school in an inner city neighborhood. She has two older brothers, ages 12 and 18. She does not see her father very often, about every 3 months. Her mother and Sashay have a very close relationship. Her mother works two part-time jobs. Sashay has been diagnosed with asthma since she was 3 years of age. She has been to the emergency room about twice a year since she was diagnosed with asthma. At times she has also been hospitalized and treated for pneumonia. She has become afraid of entering the hospital through the emergency room. However, once she is in the ER she calms down and interacts well with the medical staff. Here longest hospitalization was for 5 days when she battled pneumonia when she was in kindergarten.

Sashay has allergies, primarily to dust and mold. Living in older apartment homes and residing with an older brother who occasionally smokes at home has at times exacerbated her asthma. Dust and mold can trigger her allergies, which present as a runny nose and cough which, in turn, can cause her asthma symptoms to flare up. Sashay has weekly appointments for allergy shots and takes medication as necessary to treat her allergies. Addressing her brother's smoking in the home has been attempted, but her mother's pleas for him to smoke outside the apartment have met with limited success.

Sashay makes good grades at school. She is an especially proficient reader, with good reading comprehension. She enjoys reading in front of the class. She has several friends in her classroom and these girls interact regularly at weekly Girl Scout meetings. They also regularly have play dates after school and on weekends. Sashay is described by her mother as a "happy" child with a positive outlook on her life. She typically is "sunny" and outgoing. She is able to "speak up" for herself and stand her ground when engaging in normal sibling battles. She is likely to state her opinion and argue her views in a very positive manner and her good verbal abilities and good skills for expressing her emotions contribute to her positive emotional adjustment. Thus, she copes well and is functioning well in all areas of her life.

The exception to this is coping with emergency room visits. Sashay has had negative experiences in the ER in the past where she has needed IV administration of fluids and had to have steroid shots because she was very congested related to allergies, asthma, or pneumonia. She becomes very agitated, with rapid shallow breathing, upon entry into the ER. Her reactions do not generalize to treatments at the doctor's office. Her mother describes Sashay's behavior as being as "good as gold" in this setting. This is interesting because Sashay has had breathing treatments and shots on an emergency basis in the doctor's office as well as in the ER. There is one other issue for the health professional to address and this is infrequent use of her inhaler at school. Sashay is apt to forget to use her inhaler during the school day. Moreover, it is often missing when she needs to use it to the playground.

In order to address Sashay's issues her pediatrician has referred her for consultation with the health educator connected to the medical practice. This health educator has a master's degree in community health. After graduating, the health educator, who completed internship experiences with the asthma team and other medical teams at the local children's hospital, developed her consultation firm, Kid's First, designed to work with children and their parents. The health educator met Sashay's mother during her medical visit and discussed next steps to address school issues and medical fears. The health educator asked Sashay's mother and then Sashay about reasons for her not using her inhaler. One reason for not using it was embarrassment over other children watching her use it. The health educator made a trip to Sashay's classroom and explained to her classmates why the inhaler was important and how it helped Sashay. After this, her embarrassment decreased and peer support and encouragement helped her to use her inhaler in the classroom. While at the school, the health educator met with Sashay and the school nurse and during this team meeting she demonstrated appropriate use of the inhaler for Sashay.

Not having her inhaler on hand was a more difficult issue to resolve. The health educator initiated a conference with the school nurse and teacher via Skype. During this meeting they developed a written care plan for Sashay's records that demonstrated her need to keep her inhaler with her. The health educator networked with the pediatrician to get a note for the school records supporting the need for keeping an inhaler with Sashay at all times during the school day. This documentation was necessary to facilitate the use of her inhaler as needed during the school day.

At first, this plan was not successful. Sashay's mother called the health educator, and she, the health educator, and Sashay talked by telephone to understand what was causing the continued issues. Sashay mentioned that her clothes did not have pockets. Her mother stated that Sashay did have clothes with pockets. However, Sashay said that she was not wearing these outfits because they were "not cool." Through further discussion the health educator helped Sashay talk about a solution with her mother. They agreed that Sashay would wear or carry a fanny pack with her inhaler it during the school day. She would wear the fanny pack on her waist on the playground. Sashay agreed to this plan if she could use her mother's pink pack with the designs on it. Her mother readily agreed to this and the health educator planned a follow-up telephone call to check on progress with Sashay's mother.

At the follow-up call, Sashay's mother reported that inhaler use was improved at school. The health educator then had an opportunity, as rapport had been established, to ask if there were other issues they could discuss. Sashay's mother mentioned her oldest brother's smoking at home as a trigger for difficulty with her asthma. The health educator provided useful websites for Sashay's mother to review with her brother. They agreed that if the websites, which featured education on the dangers of second-hand smoke, did not serve as a catalyst for her brother's behavior to change, then he would need to attend a meeting with the health educator. Alternately, they discussed him going to meet with a nurse when Sashay went to receive her allergy shots so that he could discuss the dangers of second-hand smoke with this professional.

The health educator met with Sashay and her mother at Sashay's next visit, which involved her receiving a breathing treatment for her asthma flare-up, because she had a bad cold. At this visit, Sashay discussed her significant fears of the emergency room. She was not at afraid of the breathing treatment or anything that could happen in a doctor's office visit. She indicted she was very afraid that she might have to go to the ER. After discussing her fears more, the health educator asked Sashay to rate her fears on a scale from one to seven, with one indicating very low fear and seven indicating very high fear. Sashay indicated her fear was a "10" and "way too high" to even be on the scale. After this discussion, the health educator spoke briefly with Sashay's mother and let her mother know that the intensity of Sashay's fear could be indicative of a phobia about ER visits. Her mother shared this concern, and the health educator provided referrals, with names and contact information for two local child psychologists, each of whom specialized in treating anxiety in children. Sashay's mother made an appointment with one of the psychologists. After a review of background information the psychologist indicated that Sashay did appear to have a phobia related to being seen in the ER for medical treatments. A phobia is a very intense fear of an event or object that can result in extreme anxiety or panic as well as avoidance of the feared event or object.

The psychologist recommended treatment with a systematic desensitization procedure to try to reduce Sashay's fears. The psychologist helped Sashay develop a list of all the things about the ER that she feared. Then, Sashay rated each experience on the list in terms of how much it scared her on a scale from "0," the lowest level, to "20," the highest level. The fears were written on note cards and ordered from the lowest to the highest fear. In the meantime, Sashay was learning relaxation—using deep, slow breathing and thinking about going on her favorite vacation. The fear images were paired with relaxation over a series of sessions and slowly Sashay learned to feel relaxed and less afraid when discussing ER visits. After the desensitization procedure had finished, Sashay and her mother made a trip to the ER when Sashay was well. Her mother had called staff there and arranged a visit. Sashay did not appear afraid and did not report fear at this visit. The psychologist reviewed this visit with Sashay's mother during a subsequent visit. They agreed to stop sessions for the time being, but they planned to renew sessions should Sashay indicate re-experiencing her fears or have significant fears related to going to the ER.

After working with health professionals there was improvement in using her inhaler and reduced fear related to going to the ER. The watchful eye and expertise of the pediatrician and subsequent referrals added to feelings of well-being and positive functioning for Sashay. Her medical team had plans for continued involvement as needed to help Sashay and her mother as she coped with her asthma.

Summary

This chapter reviewed critical information on diagnosing asthma and learning to manage asthma symptoms. In addition information on educational interventions was reviewed. Health educators can play a key role in helping the child and his or her caregivers develop plans to manage the child's asthma. Written care plans also may facilitate asthma management at school. Key aspects of care plans include written instructions for administration of medications, ideas for reducing or controlling the impact of asthma triggers, and ideas for how to handle an asthma attack (e.g., take medication, sit or lie down and rest, call parent). Informing peers at school about how to help a child with asthma may help the child feel a sense of "belonging" in the school setting. Children with asthma may benefit from being involved in support groups, especially in the weeks and months immediately following diagnosis. These groups can provide critical information on signs of an asthma attack, what to do to manage an asthma attack, how to identify and reduce exposure to allergy triggers, how to use an inhaler, and how to find support at school and other settings where the child is engaged in extracurricular activities.

Exercises/Review Questions

1. After reviewing the case study, develop a list of key areas for intervention for health educators.
2. What are your ideas for helping a child referred to you by a physician because he or she is not using the inhaler as needed and also using it incorrectly?
3. If you were asked to design a training session to educate teachers about helping children with asthma, what would be key components of your session? What key educational topics would you address and why?
4. If a child with asthma, who was your client, was having difficulty communicating with a coach about feeling short of breath during a soccer game how could you help?

    (a) What are your ideas for sharing information with the child's parent?
    (b) If you had a signed release of information form (a written form, which is signed by the child's parent or legal guardian and permits the health professional to talk with another individual about the child's case), showed it to the coach, and had parent permission to talk with the coach, what recommendations might you have?

(c) How would you help the child learn to advocate—in order to let others know when he or she was experiencing asthma symptoms (what are your advocacy tips for the child?)

5. Review key websites on asthma management and develop a resource list for parents of children with asthma.

   (a) Develop a list of key websites as a parent resource.
   (b) Write a paragraph discussing your tips for parents after reviewing the websites provided in your resource list.

Key Concepts

Reactive airways disease
Symptoms of an asthma attack
CARAT—Child Asthma Risk Assessment Tool
Asthma triggers
Use of an inhaler
Adherence
Side effects of steroids to manage asthma
Roaring Adventures of Puff Asthma Management Program

References

Akinbami, L. J., Moorman, J. E., Garbe, P. L., & Sondik, E. J. (2009). Status of childhood asthma in the United States, 1980–2007. *Pediatrics, 123*, S131–S145.

Akinbami, L., Moorman, J. E., Baily, C., Zahran, H. S., King, M., Johnson C. A., … Xiang Liu. (2012). *Trends in asthma prevalence, health care use, and mortality in the United States, 2001– 2010* (pp. 1–8). Bethesda, MD: National Center for Health Statistics Data Brief, Centers for Disease Control and Prevention. Retrieved November 30, 2015, from http://www.cdc.gov/nchs/data/databriefs/db94.htm.

American Academy of Allergy, Asthma, and Immunology. (2014). Childhood (pediatric) asthma, 2014. Retrieved January 5, 2015, from http://www.aaaai.org/conditions-and-treatments/conditions-a-to-z-search/Childhood-%28pediatric%29-Asthma.aspx.

Barnett, S. B., & Nurmagambetov, T. A. (2011). Costs of asthma in the United States: 2002–2007. *Journal of Allergy and Clinical Immunology, 127*, 145–152.

Bousquet, J., Mantzouranis, E., Cruz, A. A., Aït-Khaled, N., Baena-Cagnani, C. E., Bleecker, E. R., … Zuberbier, T. (2010). Uniform definition of asthma severity, control, and exacerbations: document presented for the World Health Organization Consultation on Severe Asthma. *Journal of Allergy and Clinical Immunology, 126*(5), 926–938.

Bunyavanich, S., Rifas-Shiman, S. L., Platts-Mills, T. A., Workman, L., Sordillo, J. E., Camargo, C. A., … Litonjua, A. A. (2014). Peanut, milk, and wheat intake during pregnancy is associated with reduced allergy and asthma in children. *Journal of Allergy and Clinical Immunology, 133*(5), 1373–1382.

Centers for Disease Control and Prevention (CDC, 2014). *Fast facts: Asthma*. Retrieved February 2, 2015, from http://www.cdc.gov/nchs/fastats/asthma.htm.

Centers for Disease Control and Prevention (CDC). (2011). Vital signs: Asthma prevalence, disease characteristics, and self-management education, United States, 2001–2009. *Morbidity and Mortality Weekly Report, 60*(17), 547–552.

Chen, E., Bloomberg, G. R., Fisher, E. B., & Strunk, R. C. (2003). Predictors of repeat hospitalization in children with asthma: The role of psychosocial and socioenvironmental factors. *Health Psychology, 22*, 12–18.

Cicutto, L., To, T., & Murphy, S. (2013). A randomized controlled trial of a public health nurse-delivered asthma program to elementary schools. *Journal of School Health, 83*(12), 876–884.

Clarke, S.-A., Calam, R., Morawska, A., & Sanders, M. (2013). Developing web-based Triple P 'Positive Parenting Programme' for families of children with asthma. *Child Care, Health, and Development, 40*(2), 492–497.

DuPlessis-Erickson, C., Spett, P. L., Stoltzfu-Mullett, S., Jensen, C., & Bisson-Belseth, S. (2006). The healthy learner model for student chronic condition management—Part II: The asthma initiative. *Journal of School Nursing, 22*(6), 319–329.

García-Walker, V. (2012). Factors related to emotional responses in school-aged children who have asthma. *Issues in Mental Health Nursing, 33*(7), 406–429.

Gergen, P. J., & Togias, A. (2015). Inner City Asthma. *Immunology and Allergy Clinics of North America, 35*(1), 101–114.

Guilbert, T. W., Bacharier, L. B., & Fitzpatrick, A. M. (2014). Clinical management review: Severe asthma in children. *Journal of Allergy and Clinical Immunology Practice, 2*(5), 489–500.

Horn, I. B., Mitchell, S. J., Gillespie, C. W., Burke, K. M., Godoy, L., & Teach, S. J. (2014). Randomized trial of a health communication intervention for parents of children with asthma. *Journal of Asthma, 51*(9), 989–995. doi:10.3109/02770903.2014.930881.

Horner, S. D., & Brown, A. (2014). Evaluating the effect of an asthma management intervention for rural families. *Journal of Asthma, 51*(2), 168–177. doi:10.3109/02770903.2013.855785.

McPherson, A. C., & Redsell, S. A. (2009). Factors affecting children's involvement in asthma consultations: A questionnaire survey of general practitioners and primary care nurses. *Primary Care Respiratory Journal, 18*, 15–20.

Mosnaim G., Li, H., Martin, M., Richardson, D., Belice, P. J., Avery, E., Ryan, N., ... Powell, L. (2013). The impact of peer support and mp3 messaging on adherence to inhaled corticosteroids in minority adolescents with asthma: A randomized, controlled trial. *Journal of Allergy and Clinical Immunology Practice, 1*(5), 485–493.

National Institutes of Health, National Heart, Lung, and Blood Institute. (2007). *Expert panel report: Three guidelines for the diagnosis and management of asthma.* Bethesda, MD: U.S. DHHS.

National Institutes of Health, National Heart, Lung, and Blood Institute (2014). *What is asthma?* Retrieved February 2, 2015, from http://www.nhlbi.nih.gov/health/health-topics/topics/asthma/.

Pijnenburg, M. W., Baraldi, E., Brand, P. L. P., Carlson, K.-H., Eber, E., Frischer, T., ... Carlsen, K. C. L. (2015). Task force report, ERS statement: Monitoring asthma in children. *European Respiratory Journal, 45*, 906–925. doi:10.1183/09031936.00088814.

Sandberg, S., Jarvenpaa, S., Penttinen, A., Paton, J., & McCann, D. (2004). Asthma exacerbations in children immediately following stressful life events: A Cox's hierarchical regression. *Thorax, 59*(12), 1046–1051.

Sanders, M. R. (1999). Triple P—Positive Parenting Program: Towards an empirically validated multilevel parenting and family support strategy for the prevention of behavior and emotional problems in children. *Clinical Child and Family Psychology Review, 2*, 71–90.

Sordillo, J. E., Scirica, C. V., Rifas-Shiman, S. L., Gillman, M. W., Bunyavanich, S., Camargo, C. A., ... Litonjua, A. A. (2015). Prenatal and infant exposure to acetaminophen and ibuprofen and the risk for wheeze and asthma in children. *Journal of Allergy and Clinical Immunology, 135*(2), 441–448.

Stewart, M., Letourneau, N., Masuda, J. R., Anderson, S., Cicutto, L., McGhan, S., & Watt, S. (2012). Support needs and preferences of young adolescents with asthma and allergies: "Just no one really seems to understand." *Journal of Pediatric Nursing, 27*(5), 479–490.

Turcotte, D. A., Alker, H., Chaves, E., Gore, R., & Woskie, S. (2014). Healthy homes: In-home environmental asthma intervention in a diverse urban community. *American Journal of Public Health, 104*(4), 665–671.

Wilson, C., Rapp, K. I., Jack, L., Jr., Hayes, S., Post, R., & Malveaux, F. (2015). Asthma risk profiles of children participating in an asthma education and management program. *American Journal of Health Education, 46*(1), 13–23.

Wright, L. S., & Phipatanakul, W. (2014). Environmental remediation in the treatment of allergy and asthma: Latest updates. *Current Allergy and Asthma Reports, 14*(3), 1–10.

Chapter 3
Diabetes Mellitus

Diagnosis

Type 1 Diabetes Mellitus

Type 1 diabetes mellitus involves autoimmune destruction of B cells causing insulin deficiency in the majority of cases (Johnson & Uruakpa, 2014). The pancreas does not produce the insulin needed to break down glucose to convert it to energy. Children with type 1 diabetes need periodic insulin injections to regulate their blood glucose levels (Kucera & Sullivan, 2011). The insulin does not replace the pancreatic system, and consequently children experience "fluctuations in their blood glucose throughout the day in response to time, medication, diet, and physical activity" (p. 586, Kucera & Sullivan, 2011). Insulin is necessary to control blood sugar. Insulin is a hormone, which is made in the pancreas. Insulin is needed for glucose to enter cells and for the production and storage of fat.

Children who have type 1 diabetes have had elevated blood glucose (e.g., plasma glucose greater than or equal to 200 mg/dL; Silverstein et al., 2005). They often have unexplained weight loss along with polydipsia (excessive thirst) and polyuria (large production of urine; American Diabetes Association, 2014; Silverstein et al., 2005). The weight loss occurs due to a high loss of glucose in urine and body fluids. Children may report feeling tired, have weight loss for days or weeks, may report extreme thirst, and more frequent urination. The majority of cases of type 1 diabetes are diagnosed in youth between the ages of 6 through 18 years, but this disease can be diagnosed in infants. There is no cure for type 1 diabetes. The cause of diabetes remains unknown.

© Springer International Publishing Switzerland 2016   31
L. Nabors, *Medical and Mental Health During Childhood*, Springer
Series on Child and Family Studies, DOI 10.1007/978-3-319-31117-3_3

Type 2 Diabetes Mellitus

Type 2 diabetes mellitus arises from insulin resistance and insulin levels can be normal or high. This disease involves resistance to the action of insulin. The body does not use insulin appropriately, and high levels of blood glucose can accumulate (Kucera & Sullivan, 2011). The "cause" of type 2 diabetes has not been pinpointed. Children may experience pain or numbness in extremities and experience blurry vision. Type 2 diabetes mellitus or non-insulin-dependent diabetes mellitus is related to childhood obesity. Poor nutrition, eating too many foods high in carbohydrates or sugars and fat, can be involved in the diagnosis of type 2 diabetes. Children and adults with type 2 diabetes may have an imbalance of or lack key nutrients such as chromium, lipoic acid, vanadium, magnesium, or other fatty acids.

Type 2 diabetes is often diagnosed in children who have a family history of this disease. It is often diagnosed after a period of stress, infection, or illness. In type 2 diabetes C-peptide levels are high, which is indicative of a higher than average level of insulin production and an insulin resistant state. C-peptide is a protein by-product of insulin production and is measured in blood. For type 2 diabetes insulin production may be high at first and then there is a period of insulin resistance. The pancreas works hard to produce insulin, but over time it cannot produce enough insulin. Then, blood glucose levels are not able to remain at normal levels. In order to improve outcomes medication is used and children need to eat foods that are high in fiber and whole grains. Children also may take nutritional supplements to improve the action of insulin in the body (American Diabetes Association, 2012a, 2014).

The differential diagnosis of type 1 or type 2 diabetes can be somewhat unclear and it can take time to pinpoint an accurate diagnosis (American Diabetes Association, 2012a, 2014). Type 1 diabetes and type 2 diabetes are discussed in this chapter. However, there is more of an emphasis on discussion of type 1 diabetes throughout this chapter.

Prevalence

Eight percent of the population in the United States has diabetes (Johnson & Uruakpa, 2014). Dabelea et al. (2014) provided information about the prevalence of type 1 and type 2 diabetes in children and adolescents (assessing youth 20 years or younger) in the United States. The prevalence of type 1 diabetes was 1.93 per 1,000 children. The occurrence of type 1 diabetes increased from 2001 to 2009. Dabelea et al. estimated that the incidence of this disease will keep increasing. Rates of occurrence were highest in white youth. In America, approximately 13,000 youths are diagnosed with type 1 diabetes each year (Centers for Disease Control and Prevention, 2012). Dabelea et al. reported that type 2 diabetes was occurring in 0.46 per 1,000 youth in 2009. The rate of type 2 diabetes among youth has been increasing. As mentioned, this may be related to increasing rates of obesity among children and adolescents. Type 2 diabetes is more common in black and Hispanic youth and relatively less frequent in white children.

Impact on Children

Children with Type 1 diabetes require insulin, which can be administered in a number of ways. An insulin pump (continuous subcutaneous infusion) is popular. The pump allows for the administration of shorter acting insulin; children bolus or give an extra dose of insulin at mealtimes (Soni & Ng, 2014). Children often use insulin pumps to continuously monitor glucose levels. Pumps provide periodic injections of insulin via a needle guide and cannula under the child's skin. The pump is typically worn on the child's waistband (Kucera & Sullivan, 2011). Other methods of administration include shots and insulin pens. These methods of administration typically provide more long-lasting insulin and the child also gives a bolus at meals. The bolus dose is typically of more rapid acting insulin. There is not a difference in glycemic control among the various methods of administration (e.g., pumps versus shots; Sony & Ng, 2014; Yeh et al., 2012). Pumps with sensors (continuous glucose sensors) have shown promise in offering more control of blood glucose levels and are an area for further testing and research.

Diabetes has a significant impact on children. For a child with diabetes, food is fuel. It is always important to count carbohydrates at meals and snacks. Counting the carbohydrates in foods determines insulin administration. Children are often using a diabetic insulin pump and they bolus or give themselves a dose of insulin through the pump in coordination with meals and carbohydrate consumption. Some children use the insulin pen and give themselves injections or a parent may assist younger children in giving injections. The child also has to test his or her blood sugar levels at regular intervals and when he or she feels either "high" or "low." If the child feels high or low, then testing blood sugar levels may be a way to determine whether to have a snack or administer insulin to make sure that blood glucose levels remain at acceptable levels.

Needing to test one's blood (e.g., a finger prick) and needing to eat differently can cause a child to feel conspicuous. Moreover, experiencing episodes of hyperglycemia and hypoglycemia can cause a child to feel disoriented and have to go the nurse, which also can make a child feel conspicuous. Children with diabetes may not be in school with another child who experiences this chronic illness. They may benefit from support groups or attending summer camps with other peers who have diabetes to gain peer support. It can be very stressful to need to monitor food intake, count the carbohydrates in food, and check one's blood sugar constantly. Moreover, stress and exercise are other factors that can influence blood glucose levels. Management of diabetes is complex and has long-term negative health consequences if the disease is poorly managed. Therefore, coping with this disease can be very stressful and have a large impact on the child and his or her parents or caregivers.

Assessment

Regular measurement of glycosated hemoglobin or HbA1c is a marker for diabetes management. HbA1c represents average levels of glycemic control over several months. HbA1c is strongly predictive of long-term health outcomes (including negative health outcomes) and thus is considered a gold standard in assessment. HbA1c should be assessed about every 3 months. HbA1c levels can vary. Thus, assessment of daily self-monitoring of blood glucose records, in addition to HbA1c levels, may provide better information for understanding fluctuations in diabetes management, especially if the child has type 1 diabetes. If HbA1c levels can be maintained at below or about 7 %, there is likely to be fewer medical complications (American Diabetes Association, 2014). Hackworth et al. (2013) also reported that an HbA1c assessment below 7.5 is an indicator of good control. Health educators and mental health counselors should remain aware of the child's HbA1c levels and stay in contact with the child's medical team so that they understand the child's medical needs and learn of best practices for managing the child's disease.

It also is important to examine child emotional functioning and adherence or abilities to follow the medical recommendations or to "adhere" to medical recommendations. Assessing the parent–child relationship and their ability to partner and form a team to manage the child's diabetes is another important area for questions. Finally, assessing child diet, stress levels, and exercise regimens are three key areas to learn about the child's abilities to manage his or her diabetes. The child also should be regularly monitoring his or her blood glucose levels and receiving parental support and guidance for insulin administration. Good nutrition and, if recommended by doctors, regular use of nutritional supplements should be assessed.

Disease Management

Management of type 1 diabetes involves administration of insulin given on a schedule. A bolus dosage may be delivered to correct for meals. Self-monitoring of blood glucose levels is needed. Nutrition is important and reducing or monitoring carbohydrate intake is a key component of disease management. Eating a well-balanced diet and measuring food—to ensure accurate counting of carbohydrates—may be an important part of disease management, especially for children with type 1 diabetes. Eating foods that are high in nutrient density and low in simple sugars is recommended. Regular exercise and learning how to reduce stress are other factors to address when managing diabetes (Anderson, Svoren, & Laffel, 2007; Weinzimer, Doyle, & Tamborlane, 2005). Children with type 2 diabetes often are administered Metformin or other oral medications to manage insulin levels (Copeland et al., 2013). Administration of exogenous insulin is critical for the management of diabetes, whereas children with type 2 diabetes are more likely to take medications to manage their disease. The aforementioned disease management strategies (e.g., reducing stress, eating right, and exercising) will also help with maximizing the benefits of insulin for youth with type 2 diabetes. In the first month to about a year after being diagnosed with type 1 diabetes, children may experience a honeymoon period, where blood glucose levels are fairly well controlled.

The medical management of type 1 diabetes is very complex and may involve many medical professionals, including endocrinologists and their teams as well as ancillary services including nutrition, stress management and health education, and behavioral health services (mental health counseling). Families of a child with type 1 diabetes may report significant benefit from receiving family-centered care and prefer care coordination in order to help them manage the many appointments for their child. Katz, Laffel, Perrin, and Kuhlthau (2012) examined this notion by comparing the reports of caregivers of children with type 1 diabetes to those of caregivers of children with special needs using data from National Survey of Children with Special Healthcare Needs (in 2005–2006). Caregivers, usually parents, of children with type 1 diabetes reported greater impact of their child's medical condition compared to the reports of caregivers of children with other types of healthcare needs. Katz et al. found that one-third of the caregivers of a child with type 1 diabetes reported restricting time at work and experiencing financial impact related to their child's disease. If caregivers had care coordination and family-centered care, there was less impact in terms of missed work and financial impact. Thus, increasing care coordination and offering family-centered care can be important protective factors for the family.

There are many good references available to assist children and parents in management of diabetes. One of these resources is a book by Chaloner (2013), entitled "Diabetes and Me: An Essential Guide for Children and Parents." The American Diabetes Association (ADA) is another of the many great resources for education for parents and children. The website has a section for "parents and kids" (http://www.diabetes.org/living-with-diabetes/parents-and-kids/?loc=lwd-slabnav)   that has guidelines for management at school and guidelines for everyday wisdom that offer great information on diabetes management. The ADA (2012b) has developed guidelines for management of diabetes in school and day care settings. Development of a written action plan for diabetes management can be beneficial in these settings. Ideas for what to do in terms of snacks, insulin administration, meals, and blood glucose testing should be addressed in these plans, and, of course, emergency diabetes management is a cornerstone of written plans for school.

Health Concerns. Children with type 1 diabetes may have increased weight gain or increased body mass index after being diagnosed with diabetes, especially after the honeymoon period ends (de Vries et al., 2014). Girls may have greater weight gain compared to boys. Girls may be sensitive about their weight gain and this is an issue to be monitored by the medical team. Girls may also be prone to eating disorders and not administering insulin to control their weight (Butwicka, Frisén, Almquist, Zethelius, & Lichtenstein, 2015). Interestingly, de Vries et al. (2014) found that children who were on the insulin pump for longer periods did not show as significant of a weight gain.

Various studies have shown that children tend to have poor metabolic control and do not adequately manage their treatment (e.g., Chang, Yeh, Lo, & Shih, 2007; Frey, Ellis, Templin, Naar-King, & Gutai, 2006). If their disease is not managed well, they face significant long-term health complications including visual problems (retinopathy); nerve damage (neuropathy); and renal disease, which can result in renal failure or the need for dialysis (American Diabetes Association, 2014; Buckloh et al., 2008). It is noteworthy that, irrespective of whether children have type 1 or type 2 diabetes, they face significant long-term health outcomes. Children with diabetes may face other medical problems and these include digestive problems, circulation problems, and visual impairment (Johnson & Uruakpa, 2014). They may also have increased chances for thyroid and cardiac disease (American Diabetes Association, 2014).

Children who have type 1 diabetes face several other health concerns, such as hypoglycemia and hyperglycemia, which can result in heart palpitations, nausea, rapid breathing, and various other symptoms. Children and their parents/caregivers may also be afraid of experiencing a "low" or low blood glucose levels, termed a hypoglycemic episode. When this occurs the brain can have an inadequate supply of glucose. The brain is dependent on a continuous supply of glucose from the circulation; therefore, blood to brain glucose transport is critical to survival. Thus, the dangers of a low are very real and fears of a low are common in children (American Diabetes Association, 2014). When experiencing low blood glucose levels the child can feel confused and cognitive functioning can change (Silverstein et al., 2005). Many children have behavioral changes, such as becoming irritable. During a low, the child can have difficulty paying attention and mental flexibility is decreased. The child also can experience palpitations, tremors, and headache. When experiencing a low it is important for the child to have an easily digested and absorbed carbohydrate followed by a snack with protein, as protein assists with absorption of the carbohydrates.

Hyperglycemia is also a problem for children with diabetes. A hyperglycemic episode or a "high" involves an excess of or "too much" blood glucose in the blood plasma (Cryer, Davis, & Shamoon, 2003; American Diabetes Association, 2014). There also may be glucose in the child's urine. Hyperglycemia involves needs to urinate frequently, being very thirsty or hungry, nausea/vomiting, weight loss, fatigue, and changes in mood and cognition (Kucera & Sullivan, 2011). Treatment of hyperglycemia involves the administration of insulin. If left untreated, patients could experience coma and long-term medical complications affecting the eyes, heart, kidneys, and nerves.

Diabetic ketoacidosis (DKA) results from insulin deficiency. About 30 % of children with type 1 diabetes may experience DKA and have to be hospitalized. DKA involves an accumulation of ketones in the blood (leading to metabolic acidosis). This problem can occur after children have been diagnosed, if children do not administer or "skip" insulin administration or if they experience a significant hyperglycemic episode. It can occur when the child experiences trauma or illness (Wolfsdorf et al., 2007). DKA is serious and can result in cerebral edema and can result in death. If a child is experiencing DKA, insulin is typically administered intravenously and physicians monitor insulin levels, fluids, and potassium levels (Silverstein et al., 2005). Rosenbloom (2007) reported that DKA occurs in 10–70% of children newly diagnosed with type 1 diabetes and 5–52% of those children newly diagnosed with type 2 diabetes. Increased cerebral blood flow has been found in children with DKA (Rosenbloom, 2007). Children with a history of DKA episodes, those with psychiatric problems, adolescent girls, children with family problems, and children who omit doses of insulin might be at risk for DKA episodes. Children who are using the pump can also face risk, if the delivery of short-acting insulin is interrupted (Wolfsdorf et al., 2007).

Adherence

Amed et al. (2013) found that less than 10% of children with type 1 diabetes were meeting recommended guidelines for following medical recommendations (i.e., adherence). Children who had been diagnosed with diabetes for longer than 4 years were having relatively more problems with adherence. Consistent administration of recommended insulin doses, having a healthy diet, and managing carbohydrate intake are cornerstones to good management in children with type 1 diabetes (Patton, Dolan, Chen, & Powers, 2013). Children with type 2 diabetes struggle with following medical regimens, and using charts to help them remember to take medications and improve diet can be helpful for them as well. Rewarding children for good adherence, with praise and tangible prizes (e.g., time spent with parents or extra "screen time") may provide a boost to children struggling with adherence. Not knowing how to care for one's diabetes can negatively impact adherence, and therefore education is a tool for improving adherence. Children need to learn the importance of counting carbohydrates, regularly testing their blood glucose levels, and eating healthy foods and not drinking soda with sugar in it to optimally manage their diabetes. They also need to learn about the importance of regular, moderate levels of exercise and its positive impact on diabetes (American Diabetes Association, 2014; Hood, Peterson, Rohan, & Drotar, 2009).

Several other factors may impact adherence. Feelings of depression may be negatively related to adherence in children (Hood et al., 2006; Kongkaew, Jampachaisri, Chaturongkul, & Scholfield, 2014). Experiencing life stress and anxiety also can negatively impact adherence (Herzer & Hood, 2010). It is important to assess for the severity of emotional problems, in order to support the child. On the positive side, Marrero et al. (2013) reported that if peers support children in their diabetes management it can be easier for them to reach diabetes management goals. Parent or caregiver support of the child and communication between parents and the child also are critical to good management of diabetes (Miller & Drotar, 2007). Positive communication, in terms of what the child is doing well and can do to impact positive results, may be more effective in involving children in care, thereby improving adherence.

Adolescence and the transition to becoming an adolescent is a risk period for adherence problems in children with diabetes (see Rausch et al., 2012). Health educators and counselors working with children during this key transitional period need to be conscious of potential problems in adherence during adolescence. Health professionals and other adults need to be ready to problem-solve and trouble-shoot with adolescents to help them overcome difficulties with following medical recommendations for insulin administration, diet, and other key behaviors needed to assure optimal management of diabetes.

Psychosocial and Emotional Functioning

Children with diabetes may experience more psychological problems than children who do not have this disease (Butwicka, Frisén, Almqvist, Zethelius, & Lichtenstein, 2015). For example, children who have repeated bouts of DKA may experience psychiatric problems and be at risk for emotional problems (Silverstein et al., 2005). A fifth of youth with diabetes may have two or more psychiatric disorders. Butwicka et al. reported that children with diabetes are more likely to experience problems with substance use, depression, and anxiety. Depression may be the most common mental health problem for children with diabetes, followed by anxiety (Gonzalez et al., 2008; Hackworth et al., 2013). When depression levels are significant, referral to a mental health professional with experience in diabetes management is recommended. Importantly, children who are experiencing depression may not take care of their diabetes well, and thus be at risk for poor glycemic control (Gonzalez et al., 2008). The health professional with knowledge about diabetes can also address educational issues around self-care, which could help improve feelings of self-efficacy for diabetes management.

Kucera and Sullivan (2011) conducted a review of studies examining school functioning of children with type 1 diabetes. They found that children with diabetes may experience social and emotional difficulties at school. In addition, they are more likely to face academic difficulties and miss school compared to their counterparts who do not have chronic illnesses. Children with type 1 diabetes may have more learning disabilities and cognitive problems compared to their peers. Frequent bouts of mild hypoglycemia have been associated with lower scores on tasks assessing abstract reasoning. Psycho-motor speed may be slowed and difficulties with focusing attention may be observed. The aforementioned academic problems may be exacerbated in children with poor glycemic control and/or poor diabetes management. Kucera and Sullivan recommended care plans be written for schools and they detailed key elements of such plans, including needs for testing, snacking, procedures for special events, common presentation of hypoglycemia for the child, and a communication plan (to notify the school nurse, parents, and the medical team). Education of school personnel about diabetes and its management is a front-line intervention to support the child. They recommended shared management of diabetes management at school, with the school nurse as a potential team leader and child involvement in management of his or her illness. Children should also be given space and privacy to test blood glucose levels and teachers should have snacks on hand to that children can snack if needed.

Interventions

Christie et al. (2014) evaluated the effectiveness of the Child and Adolescent Structured Competencies Approach to Diabetes Education (CASCADE) training model for children with diabetes and their families. This program, based in the UK (England), focused on training a nurse and another member of the diabetes care team to deliver training to children and families. The program is based on the notion of motivating children and parents and is also oriented toward brief, solution-focused problem-solving. There are four modules for the program: (1) learning about food, insulin, and glucose; (2) reviewing blood glucose testing (including coping with lows, highs); (3) learning about adjusting insulin; and (4) lessons for "living with diabetes." At the end of the educational modules, children and their parents/caregivers develop a blueprint for success for helping the child cope and live with his or her diabetes. This is a detailed self-management plan tailored to the needs of the individual child and family.

For this study, children between the ages of 8–16 years and their parents/caregivers received training using the abovementioned CASCADE program (Christie et al., 2014). Although there were not changes in HbA1c levels, children indicated improved confidence for managing their diabetes and wanting to try "harder" to manage their diabetes. Family relationships also improved. Christie et al. pointed out the benefits of training nurses on diabetes care teams, because the medical team was "armed" with critical information that would help the team promote diabetes management and positive coping for children for years to come. This program is relatively cost-effective in approach, and further investigation is needed to determine whether this intervention impacts child functioning in the long term or can assist children with coping and adjustment during difficult periods in adolescence.

Group interventions are a common method for educating children and adolescents with diabetes. Sharing information with peers about one's diabetes may offer support critical to positive attitudes toward illness and diabetes management. Plante and Lobato (2008) reviewed group treatments for youth with diabetes. They reported there was a positive impact for group interventions. They found educational groups and action-oriented groups did help children manage their disease. These types of groups afford children opportunities to practice skills such as goal setting, problem-solving, dietary change, developing behavioral contracts for meeting diabetes management goals, monitoring blood glucose testing, and stress management. Plante and Lobato reported that several studies used anchored instruction where leaders taught problem-solving skills "through video presentation of real-life diabetes care scenarios" (p. 99). With anchored instruction parts of the video were replayed to "… highlight clues to solve the problem" (Plante & Lobato, 2008, p. 100). Group members could problem-solve with guidance from group leaders and use different parts of the video as cues for discussion. Results for anchored instruction were positive, resulting in improved knowledge about nutrition, meal planning, and problem-solving. Plante and Lobato also reviewed the findings of eight studies focusing on teaching youth stress management skills. For these studies, education appeared to be successful in improving children's abilities to recognize and cope with personal stress. The impact of social skills training groups and two interventions to improve family functioning were successful in improving disease management.

Many of the group interventions target children. Parents of children with diabetes also may encounter significant stress and uncertainty, such that they too might benefit from support groups. Hoff et al. (2005) discovered that groups for parents of children newly diagnosed with diabetes showed promise for decreasing parent stress and improving child behaviors. For their intervention, parents received training to minimize feelings of uncertainty and distress. Parents learned techniques for managing feelings of uncertainty as well as learning problem-solving and communication skills.

Parents may have free time as their children attend groups to promote diabetes management. Groups for parents can be conducted at the same time as children's groups. At key intervals, perhaps after three or four sessions, parents and children could attend joint groups to share experiences and work on family problem-solving and communication skills. Conducting support groups for both parents and children may ease distress and improve knowledge, leading to improvements in parent and child feelings of self-efficacy for management of the child's diabetes. In addition, joint groups, with parents and children, can foster the teamwork approach and group facilitators or leaders can espouse a team approach, with parents guiding and praising child efforts at self-management.

The internet may be an avenue for supporting youth. For example, several researchers in the TEENCOPE study group examined the effectiveness of two internet interventions for youth with type 1 diabetes (Grey et al., 2013). Participants were between the ages of 11 and 14 years. Each program provided five lessons for youth transitioning to adolescence. The first intervention—TEENCOPE group—used ethnically diverse characters to deliver messages about problem-solving, stress management, being positive (i.e., using positive self-talk), and conflict resolution. Adolescents communicated through a monitored discussion board. Over half of the youth in this group participated in the discussion boards. The other group—Managing Diabetes group—considered a control condition, delivered messages about healthy eating, physical activity, monitoring blood glucose, and self-management. In this group, participants could follow links to gain access to more complex information.

Three hundred and twenty youth with type 1 diabetes were assigned to the two groups (mean HbA1c for the youth was approximately 8.4; Grey et al., 2013). There were relatively few differences in performance on outcome measures between the TEENCOPE and Managing Diabetes groups. Many of the youth attended a majority of the sessions. After assessing outcomes, youth could "cross-over" and participate in the other group. Youth who participated in both interventions had better health outcomes compared to youth who participated in only one of the interventions. Perceptions of stress, family conflict, social acceptance, quality of life, and perceived stress improved when adolescents participated in both groups, and there was a trend for improvements in HbA1c levels for youth who went through both programs. The researchers evaluating this project surmised that the Managing Diabetes intervention assisted in improving primary engagement coping with the disease, while the TEENCOPE program aided in secondary engagement coping—coping with stress, dealing with emotions, etc. The researchers noted that youth from low-income families were less likely to volunteer to participate in the groups, and therefore, more culturally appropriate interventions may need to be designed for these youth (Grey et al., 2013).

Quirk, Blake, Tennyson, Randell, and Glazebrook (2014) reviewed the effectiveness of physical activity for youth (age 18 or younger) in 26 studies. The majority of the studies ($n = 24$) reported at least one positive health outcome for youth participating in exercise. Many of the studies found positive change in blood glucose levels and improvements in body mass index. Exercise or physical activity sessions with youth ranged from 30 to 120 min, with more recent studies having sessions of 60 min or less. Interventions lasted from 2 to 39 weeks, which is a fairly large difference in the "dose" of the intervention. Interventions focused on aerobic activities (e.g., swimming, running, or dance) or aerobic and strengthening activities. In some studies, advice was provided about insulin, making the interventions multi-faceted. Thus, it is hard to untangle which parts of the intervention and what dose is "most" helpful and this remains an area for further study. Only 4 of the studies examined the relationship between engaging in physical activity and change in children's reports of quality of life. Quirk and colleagues recommended examining this link as an area for future research. It was evident that results were positive suggesting that coaching children and supporting their engagement in physical activity is a frontline intervention for children with diabetes. Because exercise can influence blood glucose levels, it is advisable that health professionals recommend engaging in increased levels of mild to moderate physical activity along with continued monitoring of blood glucose levels.

Exercise, specifically aerobic activity, and dietary intervention can lower HbA1c levels in individuals with type 2 diabetes. Andrews et al. (2011) presented information on the effectiveness of a randomized controlled trial examining care as usual, a dietary regimen, and an exercise plus dietary intervention. Individuals in this study were between 30 and 80 years of age; however, the interventions and principal ideas of this study are applicable for children. The diet regimen aimed to help participants lose 5–10 % of their bodyweight. Guidance was provided to participants about portion size and they received coaching about how to select foods with lower energy density, fat content, and lower glycemic index scores. Dieticians interviewed patients and assisted them in setting goals Dieticians and nurses worked with participants to set goals each week and provided advice about diet to participants. Those participating in the diet plus activity group also were asked to do brisk walking for at least 30 min for 5 days per week. When evaluating the impact of the interventions, Andrews et al. reported that the dietary intervention was successful and resulted in improved HbA1c levels, improved use of diabetes medications, and improvements in weight loss. Adding physical activity as an intervention did not result in additional improvements in health outcomes when compared to the dietary intervention. Insulin resistance and HbA1c levels worsened in the usual care group, which served as the comparison group. Perhaps the exercise did not impact key variables related to health outcomes because the dose or amount of exercise was weak or not strong enough to influence health outcomes.

The American Diabetes Association implemented a school-based program to prevent type 2 diabetes in school-age children (Valde, 2011). This educational program was based on the notion that obesity is a strong risk factor for type 2 diabetes in children. Obesity, in turn, is also related to low levels of physical activity and poor nutrition. Diabetes prevention programs promote healthy eating and exercise for youth and their families. This includes encouraging participants to eat low calorie, nutrient dense foods and reduce consumption of high calorie, high fat foods. Portion control—and not being supersized, in terms of what children eat—can be another key ingredient in prevention programs. Drinking fewer sodas with sugar and eating fewer high calorie snacks are also reviewed in prevention programs. Reducing screen time and increasing physical activity levels are key ingredients to obesity prevention and the prevention of type 2 diabetes. The aforementioned information was critical to the development and implementation of a diabetes prevention program delivered in elementary schools (Valde, 2011).

The American Diabetes Association worked with local schools to implement a diabetes prevention program (Valde, 2011). They involved the physical education teacher at the school and the program was offered in physical education classes for third and fourth grade students. Children learned information about healthy lifestyles and ideas about prevention of type 2 diabetes. They also learned about type 1 diabetes. The impact of exercise and healthy eating on management of type 2 diabetes was emphasized. A pretest and posttest was use to examine child knowledge about nutrition and how to prevent type 1 and type 2 diabetes. A 24 % increase in student knowledge level was recorded in schools participating in the intervention. Informal feedback from the students also heralded the success of the program. Due to the program's success, volunteers planned to implement the program in elementary schools that did not participate in the intervention. Strong community partnerships that provided a solid foundation of support for implementing the program and support from volunteers to implement program activities in schools were keys to the program's success (Valde, 2011).

Roles for Health Educators

There are many interventions aimed to improve diabetes management and health outcomes for individuals with diabetes. However, more interventions with children are needed. Long-term follow-up on the impact of these interventions will provide information about whether early intervention is a protective factor for youth, enabling them to do better in terms of management during adolescence and beyond. Similarly, less is known about how to tailor interventions to make them culturally relevant (Mc Manus & Savage, 2010). In order to adapt interventions, manuals may need to be translated into other languages or interventions may need to be delivered with the assistance of professional interpreters. Those delivering interventions also may need training to understand the culture of study participants. Surveys to examine health outcomes, such as self-efficacy for disease management and family functioning, may need to be administered by research assistants who are culturally competent (Mc Manus & Savage, 2010).

Shared decision-making with parents/caregivers and parent support and monitoring is important (Silverstein et al., 2005; Yeh et al., 2012). As the child matures, parents/caregivers may need to renegotiate their roles and the child may need to assume a greater role in self-management of eating, exercising, and insulin administration. Teaching parents and children to remain flexible as diabetes management roles shift is an important contribution as the child grows and parent and child management roles change. It also is important to remind parents that insulin levels may increase during puberty (Yeh et al., 2012).

Goal setting with children and parents/caregivers is an effective intervention for assisting the child to reach diabetes management goals (Soni & Ng, 2014). The health educator can ensure that members of the child's medical team are "on the same page" in terms of goals for diabetes management. After confirming the team's goals for the child, the health educator can educate the child and parent about these goals. Self-monitoring, by recording glucose levels when testing and recording carbohydrates in snacks and meals, is one method for tracking progress. This information can be used by the medical team to determine how the child is progressing toward meeting his or her goals. Moreover, the information is useful to parents and the child as they monitor the child's progress on a daily and weekly basis. It may be advantageous to reward the child for monitoring (i.e., keeping records on a chart), in order to reinforce the child for recording his or her progress. Then, praise and perhaps other rewards can be provided when the child has positive or lower blood glucose levels or has improved the "health" level of his or her eating. The last section of this chapter presents information using a case study that illustrates areas for intervention and roles for health educators.

Case Study

Jenny is a 10-year-old girl who was diagnosed with type 1 diabetes in the past 2 months. She is overweight. However, she had recently lost weight and was urinating very frequently. Jenny also reported feeling tired and was asking to take naps often. This caused her aunt, whom she was staying with for the summer, to worry about her health and bring her to see a pediatrician, who made an initial diagnosis of type 1 diabetes. After this, the pediatrician referred Jenny for care at the local children's hospital. The hospital has a childhood diabetes team comprised of endocrinologists, nurses, diabetes educators, a child psychologist, and a health educator.

After a visit, the medical team learned more about Jenny's history. Jenny was residing with her aunt over the summer, but this may become permanent, pending a court decision. Jenny experienced periods of homeless in Atlanta, her home. She has also been in and out of care with different family relatives. Her mother has had difficulties with substance use. Her mother does not have a house and Jenny and her mother and younger sister have been residing in hotels and shelters. She has not attended school regularly and is behind a grade due to missing school so frequently. Her mother brought Jenny to a Child and Family Services Unit in Atlanta to find her a case worker, because she was worried about Jenny's health. It was her mother who actually suggested Jenny visit her aunt for the summer. Upon uncovering the history of neglect and lack of housing and food, the caseworker in Atlanta opened a court case. A judge will decide if Jenny remains in her mothers' care, her aunt's care, or goes to live with another relative. Jenny's aunt has temporary custody over the summer. The case worker for Child and Family Services is her guardian until the judge can make a decision about long-term placement for Jenny.

Jenny's aunt is just learning about type 1 diabetes in children. She has begun administering insulin and provides doses on a regular basis. Jenny's HbA1c level is around 7, which is good. Her aunt remains concerned that Jenny's mother will not be able to administer insulin regularly nor will she be able to help Jenny watch her carbohydrate intake. In Atlanta, the family diet is mostly carbohydrates and is high in refined sugar. Soda with sugar is a drink of choice rather than water or milk. Meals are infrequent and the children often overeat at a meal, because they are not sure when the next meal will be. The endocrinologist at the children's hospital has recommended that insulin be administered by an adult using an insulin pen, as Jenny has a history of misusing medications and her aunt expressed fear about using the pump to administer insulin. The endocrinologist has recommended consultation with the child psychologist who works with the diabetes team. He also recommended enrolling Jenny and her aunt in the buddy and education programs at the hospital.

Jenny is enrolled in a support group with other children who have type 1 diabetes at her local children's hospital. She has gone to one session and gotten to know the group leaders, a health educator and a child psychologist. Jenny is very personable and the group leaders believe she will do very well in the group, which is comprised of three other children who are enrolled in elementary school. The group is focused on helping children learn to count their carbohydrates, eat more vegetables and fruits, and exercise regularly. Parents or caregivers meet with the health educator and receive pamphlets to learn what children are reviewing in the groups. The health educator is assigning Jenny's aunt a buddy, who is another mother of a child who has been coping with diabetes for a few years. This mother is a volunteer for the buddy program sponsored by the diabetes team. Jenny and her aunt also were referred, by the health educator, to a pediatric dietician at the children's hospital.

The child psychologist on the team is going to interview Jenny to determine if she would benefit from counseling, given the turbulent nature of her developmental history in Atlanta. The child psychologist has been in contact with the case worker in Atlanta and Jenny's mother to gather historical information prior to her meeting with Jenny. During the meeting with Jenny, the child psychologist plans to screen for intellectual functioning. The child psychologist plans to talk with Jenny's aunt to determine if educational testing, regarding appropriate placement for the next academic year, will be required.

The health educator and child psychologist will meet to determine a case lead for the diabetes team. One of these two professionals will be the lead on the case and organize follow-up visits and care for Jenny. This care manager will provide information to the case manager in Atlanta, will determine if Jenny has improved knowledge about her diabetes and its management, is functioning adequately – in terms of emotional functioning – and has had adequate assessment of academic abilities. This is important as Jenny needs to "catch up" on missed educational opportunities. It is hoped that this will occur during the summer through tutoring. This case study highlights roles for both the health educator and a psychologist to add to the medical management of the child's disease and to contribute to child well-being.

Summary

This chapter reviewed critical information on the management of type 1 diabetes and type 2 diabetes. Material relevant to improving child adherence and functioning was presented. Information about interventions to improve child functioning was emphasized. The case study illustrated roles for health educators and psychologists. Currently, the cause and cure for diabetes remains unknown. This disease impacts many youth and their families, and finding a cure will help many. Improving medical management of this disease is critical, as improved medical management, in terms of reducing stress, improving healthy eating, exercising, administering insulin (type 1 diabetes), and taking medications (type 2 diabetes), remains critical tasks for improving health outcomes for children.

Exercises/Review Questions

1. Define type 1 and type 2 diabetes.
2. What are "best practices" for the management of type 1 diabetes in children?
3. What are possible long-term health consequences related to diabetes for children?
4. Is physical activity a cornerstone for diabetes management in your opinion? Why or why not?

   The five questions below are based on your review of the case study...

1. If you were the team leader for the hospital-based children's education group, what topics would be covered to educate children about diabetes?
2. What type of information about diabetes management should be transmitted to Jenny's aunt, and if necessary, her case worker in Atlanta?

3. How would you recommend monitoring adherence to blood glucose monitoring and insulin administration at Jenny's aunt's home over the remainder of the summer months?
4. Jenny is in the honeymoon period. How would you explain this phenomenon to her aunt?
5. How should Jenny's mother be involved, if she comes to visit Jenny over the summer months?

Key Concepts

Type 1 diabetes
Type 2 diabetes
Hyperglycemia
Hypoglycemia
Counting carbohydrates
Blood glucose testing
Insulin Pump
Glycosated hemoglobin or HbA1c
Long-term health concerns for children with diabetes
Diabetic ketoacidosis (DKA)
Emotions and diabetes
Shared management or teamwork approach to diabetes management
CASCADE training model
TEENCOPE Program

References

Amed, S., Nuernberger, K., McCrea, P., Reimer, K., Krueger, H., Aydede, S. K., … Collet, J. P. (2013). Adherence to clinical practice guidelines in the management of children, youth, and young adults with type 1 diabetes: A prospective population cohort study. *Journal of Pediatrics, 163*(2):543–548. doi:10.1016/j.jpeds.2013.01.070.
American Diabetes, A. (2014). Standards of medical care in diabetes—2014. *Diabetes Care, 37*(Supplement 1), S14–S80.
American Diabetes Association (ADA). (2012a). *Medical management of type 2 diabetes.* Alexandria, VA: American Diabetes Association.
American Diabetes Association (ADA). (2012b). Diabetes care in the school and day care setting. *Diabetes Care, 35*(Supplement 1), S76–S80. doi:10.2337/dc12-s076.
Anderson, B. J., Svoren, B., & Laffel, L. (2007). Initiatives to promote effective self-care skills in children and adolescents with diabetes mellitus. *Disease Management and Health Outcomes, 15*, 101–108.
Andrews, R. C., Cooper, A. R., Montgomery, A. A., Norcross, A. J., Peters, T. J., Sharp, D. J., … Dayan, C. M. (2011). Diet or diet plus physical activity versus usual care in patients with newly diagnosed type 2 diabetes: The early ACTID randomized controlled trial. *Lancet, 378*, 129–139.
Buckloh, L. M., Lochrie, A. S., Antal, H., Milkes, M. A., Atilio Canas, J., Hutchinson, S., & Wysocki, T. (2008). Diabetes complications in youth: Qualitative analysis of parents'

perspectives of family learning and knowledge. *Diabetes Care, 31*(8), 1516–1520. doi:10.2337/dc07-2349.

Butwicka, A., Frisén, L., Almqvist, C., Zethelius, B., & Lichtenstein, P. (2015). Risks of psychiatric disorders and suicide attempts in children and adolescents with type 1 diabetes: A population-based cohort study. *Diabetes Care, 38*(3), 453–459. doi:10.2337/dc14-0262.

Centers for Disease Control and Prevention (2012*). Children and diabetes*. Retrieved May 9, 2013, from http://www.cdc.gov/diabetes/projects/cda2.htm.

Chaloner, K. (2013). *Diabetes and me: An essential guide for children and parents*. New York, NY: Hill and Wang.

Chang, C.-W., Yeh, C.-H., Lo, F.-S., & Shih, Y.-L. (2007). Adherence behaviors in Taiwanese children and adolescents with type 1 diabetes mellitus. *Journal of Nursing and Healthcare of Chronic Illness in association with Journal of Clinical Nursing, 16*(7b), 207–214.

Christie, D., Thompson, R., Sawtell, M., Allen, E., Cairns, J., Smith, F., … Viner, R. (2014). Structured, intensive education maximizing engagement, motivation and long-term change for children and young people with diabetes: A cluster randomized controlled trial with integral process and economic evaluation–the CASCADE study. *Health Technology Assessment, 18*(20), 1–202. doi:10.3310/hta18200.

Copeland, K.C., Silverstein, J., Moore, K.R., Prazar, G.E., Raymer, T., Shiffman, R.N., … Flinn, S.K. (2013). Management of newly diagnosed type 2 diabetes mellitus (T2DM) in children and adolescents. American Academy of Pediatrics (AAP) Clinical Practice Guideline. *Pediatrics, 131*, 364–382. doi:10.1542/peds.2012-3494. Retrieved June 8, 2015, from http://www.guideline.gov/content.aspx?id=39539.

Cryer, P. E., Davis, S. N., & Shamoon, H. (2003). Hypoglycemia in diabetes. *Diabetes Care, 26*(6), 1902–1912.

Dabelea, D., Mayer-Davis, E. J., Saydah, S., Imperatore, G., Linder, B., Divers, J., … Hamman, R. F. (2014). Prevalence of type 1 and type 2 diabetes among children and adolescents from 2001 to 2009. *Journal of the American Medical Association, 311*(17), 1778–1786.

de Vries, L., Bar-Niv, M., Lebenthal, Y., Tenenbaum, A., Shalitin, S., Lazar, L., … Phillip, M. (2014). Changes in weight and BMI following the diagnosis of type 1 diabetes in children and adolescents. *Acta Diabetologica, 51*(3), 395–402.

Frey, M. A., Ellis, D., Templin, T., Naar-King, S., & Gutai, J. P. (2006). Diabetes management and metabolic control in school-age children with type 1 diabetes. *Children's Health Care, 35*, 349–363.

Gonzalez, J. S., Peyrot, M., McCarl, L. A., Collins, E. M., Serpa, L., Mimiaga, M. J., & Safren, S. A. (2008). Depression and diabetes treatment nonadherence: A meta-analysis. *Diabetes Care, 31*(12), 2398–2403.

Grey, M., Whittemore, R., Sangchoon, J., Murphy, K., Faulkner, M. S., & Delamater, A; TEENCOPE Study Group. (2013). Internet psycho-education programs improve outcomes in youth with type 1 diabetes. *Diabetes Care, 36*, 2475–2482.

Hackworth, N. J., Hamilton, V. E., Moore, S. M., Northam, E. A., Bucalo, Z., & Cameron, F. J. (2013). Predictors of diabetes self-care, metabolic control, and mental health in youth with type 1 diabetes. *Australian Psychologist, 48*, 360–368.

Herzer, M., & Hood, K. K. (2010). Anxiety symptoms in adolescents with T 1 diabetes: Association with blood glucose monitoring and glycemic control. *Journal of Pediatric Psychology, 35*(4), 415–425. doi:10.1093/jpepsy/jsp063.

Hoff, A. L., Mullins, L. L., Gillaspy, S. R., Page, M. C., Van Pelt, J. C., & Chaney, J. M. (2005). An intervention to decrease uncertainty and distress among parents of children newly diagnosed with diabetes: A pilot study. *Families, Systems, and Health, 23*(3), 329–342. doi:10.1037/1091-7527.23.3.329.

Hood, K. K., Huestis, S., Maher, A., Butler, D., Volkening, L., & Laffel, L. (2006). Depressive symptoms in children and adolescents with type 1 diabetes association with diabetes-specific characteristics. *Diabetes Care, 29*(6), 1389–1391.

Hood, K. K., Peterson, C. M., Rohan, J. M., & Drotar, D. (2009). Association between adherence and glycemic control in pediatric type 1 diabetes: a meta-analysis. *Pediatrics, 124*(6), e1171–e1179. doi:10.1542/peds.2009-0207.

Johnson, M. K., & Uruakpa, F. (2014). Comparing health impairments in special health care needs children with and without diabetes. *Universal Journal of Public Health, 2*(1), 17–24. doi:10.13189/ujph.2014.020103.

Katz, M. L., Laffel, L. M., Perrin, J. M., & Kuhlthau, K. (2012). Impact of type 1 diabetes mellitus on the family is reduced with the medical home, care coordination, and family-centered care. *Journal of Pediatrics, 160*, 861–867. doi:10.1016/j.jpeds.2011.10.010.

Kongkaew, C., Jampachaisri, K., Chaturongkul, C. A., & Scholfield, C. N. (2014). Depression and adherence to treatment in diabetic children and adolescents: A systematic review and meta-analysis of observational studies. *European Journal of Pediatrics, 173*(2), 203–212. doi:10.1007/s00431-013-2128-y.

Kucera, M., & Sullivan, A. L. (2011). The educational implications of type 1 diabetes mellitus: A review of research and recommendations for school psychological practice. *Psychology in the Schools, 48*(6), 587–603. doi:10.1002/pits.20573.

Marrero, D. G., Ard, J., Delamater. A. M., Peragallo-Dittko, V., Mayer-Davis, E. J., Nwankwo, R., & Fisher, E.B. (2013). Twenty-first century behavioral medicine: A context for empowering clinicians and patients with diabetes: A consensus report. *Diabetes Care, 36*(2), 463–470. doi:10.2337/dc12-2305.

Mc Manus, V., & Savage, E. (2010). Cultural perspectives of interventions for managing diabetes and asthma in children and adolescents from minority groups. *Child: Care, Health and Development, 36*(5), 612–622. doi:10.1111/j.365-2214.2010.01101.x.

Miller, V., & Drotar, D. (2007). Decision-making competence and adherence to treatment in adolescents with diabetes. *Journal of Pediatric Psychology, 32*(2), 178–188. doi:10.1093/jpepsy/jsj122.

Patton, S. R., Dolan, L. M., Chen, M., & Powers, S. W. (2013). Dietary adherence and mealtime behaviors in young children with type 1 diabetes on intensive insulin therapy. *Journal of the Academy of Nutrition and Dietetics, 113*(2), 258–262. doi:10.1016/j.jand.2012.09.013.

Plante, W. A., & Lobato, D. J. (2008). Psychosocial group interventions for children and adolescents with type 1 diabetes: The state of the literature. *Children's Health Care, 37*, 93–111. doi:10.1080/02739610701601361.

Quirk, H., Blake, H., Tennyson, R., Randell, T. L., & Glazebrook, C. (2014). Physical activity interventions in children and young people with type 1 diabetes mellitus: A systematic review with meta-analysis. *Diabetic Medicine, 31*(10), 1163–1173.

Rausch, J. R., Hood, K. K., Delamater, A., Pendley, J. S., Rohan, J. M., Reeves, G., … Drotar, D. (2012). Changes in treatment adherence and glycemic control during the transition to adolescence in type 1 diabetes. *Diabetes Care, 35*(6), 1219–1224.

Rosenbloom, A. L. (2007). Hyperglycemic crises and their complications in children. *Journal of Pediatric Endocrinology and Metabolism, 20*(1), 5–18.

Silverstein, J., Klingensmith, G., Copeland, K., Plotnick, L., Kaufman, F., Laffel, L., … Clark, N. (2005). Care of children and adolescents with type 1 diabetes a statement of the American Diabetes Association. *Diabetes Care, 28*(1), 186–212.

Soni, A., & Ng, S. M. (2014). Intensive diabetes management and goal setting are key aspects of improving metabolic control in children and young people with type 1 diabetes mellitus. *World Journal of Diabetes, 5*(6), 877–881. doi:10.4239/wjd.v5.i6.877.

Valde, J. G. (2011). Community program to prevent diabetes in school children. *Journal of Community Health Nursing, 28*, 215–222. doi:10.1080/07370016.2011.615183.

Weinzimer, S. A., Doyle, E. A., & Tamborlane, W., Jr. (2005). Disease management in the young diabetic patient: Glucose monitoring, coping skills, and treatment strategies. *Clinical Pediatrics, 44*, 393–403.

Wolfsdorf, J., Craig, M. E., Daneman, D., Dunger, D., Edge, J., Warren Lee, W. R., … Hanas, R. (2007). Diabetic ketoacidosis. *Pediatric diabetes, 8*(1), 28–43.

Yeh, H. C., Brown, T. T., Maruthur, N., Ranasinghe, P., Berger, Z., Suh, Y. D., … Golden, S. H. (2012). Comparative effectiveness and safety of methods of insulin delivery and glucose monitoring for diabetes mellitus: a systematic review and meta-analysis. *Annals of Internal Medicine, 157*(5), 336–347.

Chapter 4
Coping with Pain

Defining Pain in Children

In primary care and hospital settings injuries are the most common medical problem and cause of pain in children. If acute pain due to injury is not treated, it can have long-lasting effects for children. Walco (2008) defined pain (or nociception) as, "Nociception refers to the excitation of peripheral afferent neurons in response to a noxious stimulus" (p. S126). Nociception is sensory stimulation which sends a message to the brain, and pain is the subjective response to the stimulation. Thus, pain is what hurts when we respond to a noxious stimulus or injury. One good resource for learning about pain is information posted by the National Institute of Neurological Disorders and Stroke (http://www.ninds.nih.gov/disorders/chronic_pain/detail_chronic_pain.htm, 2015). At this site there is information on recent pain research, mostly focusing on adults, but the information about the pain response and transmission of pain in the nervous system is applicable for children as well.

Children typically describe pain in terms of its (1) unpleasantness; (2) its sensory attributes, such as strength, quality (throbbing, sharp); (3) location; and (4) duration (McGrath, 1990). Chronic pain lasts for more than 3 months; this can be termed "recurrent" and long-term pain (Eccleston et al., 2012). This recurring pain usually interferes with a child's daily functioning. Acute pain is usually of short duration. It is typically produced by a well-defined pain stimulus, such as an injury or a medical procedure.

There are two other types of pain that might be helpful to define. Some children may have referred pain. Referred pain may be defined as pain felt at one place or site on the body that originates from an injury or noxious stimulus at another site in the body. Another type of pain is causalgia pain. This is pain that is produced by stimuli that would normally be considered to be "nonpainful" stimuli or stimuli that do not produce pain in most children.

Children who have chronic illnesses may report experiencing pain that is not explained by their disease alone (Bromberg, Schechter, Nurko, Zempsky, &

© Springer International Publishing Switzerland 2016
L. Nabors, *Medical and Mental Health During Childhood*, Springer
Series on Child and Family Studies, DOI 10.1007/978-3-319-31117-3_4

Schanberg, 2014). That is, they may experience pain without any functional or physical cause. Thus, it is important to consider psychological and social causes of pain, in addition to physical causes. It may be that children with some chronic conditions, such as arthritis or sickle cell disease, may begin to experience disordered sensory processing that impairs the physical mechanisms by which they experience pain. Children with this type of nonfunctional pain may have "hypersensitive" sensory or nociceptive or pain systems in their bodies. These types of pain can be termed functional pain, which may be defined as, "…pain that exists without an underlying biochemical or anatomical abnormality" (p. 211; Bromberg et al., 2014).

Pain is subjective and individualized. Therefore, each child should define his or her pain as "what hurts" (McGrath, 1990). There is a subjective component to children's pain and it is crucial to assess each child's symptoms on an individual basis and design pain management strategies that work best for the child. Pain can be defined in terms of its intensity, quality, cause, and duration. There are multiple causes for pain, including mechanical, thermal, electrical, and chemical causes. For example, a thermal cause for pain might be a burn injury. A fall from a tractor could cause mechanical pain. Children may describe their pain intensity from being weak to strong. Quality descriptors for pain include terms such as aching, throbbing, tearing, and burning. Duration can encompass many descriptors that include frequency of the pain ("I'm in pain all the time; I'm in pain once in a while when it rains") and how long (how many days, months, years) the child has been experiencing pain.

Pain messages are transmitted in the child's body through the nociceptive system. Describing the pain system to children is important, because they need to understand how pain messages are transmitted in the body to comprehend how psychosocial pain management strategies can be helpful tools for reducing their pain experiences. The health educator might not need to use the term nociceptive system or explain the role of axons in transmitting pain, but a developmentally appropriate explanation of how pain messages are transmitted is critical for children. One example of an explanation for how pain messages travel in the body is presented in Fig. 4.1.

Pain messages are delivered electronically. Nociceptive processing occurs when our sensory system detects a noxious stimulus and transmits this message, via axons in the body, to the brain (McGrath, 1990; Melzak & Wall, 1965). The child's brain interprets the pain message. The pain message begins at the dendrites of primary neurons, which are peripheral nerves that synapse or connect to secondary neurons in the dorsal horn of the spinal chord (pain messages moving through this circuitry are said to move through the spinothalamic tract). The nociceptive afferents are the axons of primary neurons that take messages to the brain. Different nociceptive afferents (axons of the primary neurons) are sensitive to different types of pain. The pain message moves out from the dorsal horn, via projection neurons, whose axons extend to the brain. The spinothalamic tract is the most fundamental pathway for pain messages.

The brain then receives the pain message and interprets it. The brain can thus "act" on pain messages, lessening their impact. Once the child can grasp this concept it may be easier for him or her to follow the logic behind the notion of using

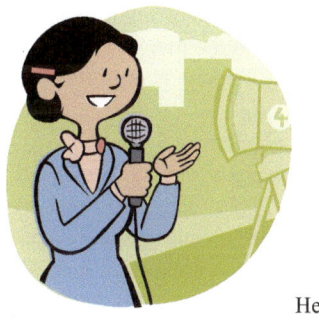

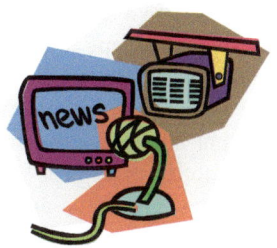

Here is how pain works.

The receptors for pain are located in many places, like the skin, muscles, bones and joints. Your arthritis can cause pain messages to start in your joints.

The A-Delta and C nerve fibers will send the pain message and then neurons will turn the pain message into an electrical signal that tells your brain you HURT. What happens is that the A and C fibers take the message up the spinothalamic track to your brain, in places called the thalamus and the frontal cortex. Your brain helps tell you about the pain message.

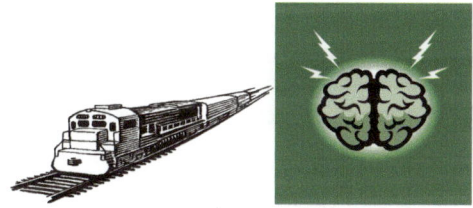

Draw a track from one of your painful joints to your brain right here.

Fig. 4.1 How pain works

mental strategies and other behavioral strategies to help him or her manage pain. It is also critical to explain to the child that the brain can make its own pain suppressors, and release endorphins, which may lessen the child's experience of pain. This has been a cursory review of how pain works for children. But, even a simple explanation, such as the one that is presented in Fig. 4.1, can help the child to grasp that his or her thinking processes and behaviors can help impact the pain experience.

Prevalence

Acute pain is the most common type of pain in children, followed by recurrent pain with no known cause (Hermann & Blanchard, 2002). Headache pain is very common in children. For instance, pediatric migraine occurs in 3–10 % of children and adolescents (Hermann & Blanchard, 2002). Arguably, an area of key importance for children is chronic pain related to medical conditions and the majority of this chapter will focus on a discussion of chronic pain related to medical conditions and the treatment of this type of pain. Headache is a frequently studied area in children's chronic pain and thus also will be referenced in this chapter.

Prevalence rates for pain experiences for children vary across studies and across type of chronic medical condition (King et al., 2011). For example, Weiss et al. (2013) reported that 11–38 % of children may experience chronic pain at some time in their lives. Headache and abdominal pain are the most common types of pain reported by children (Eccleston et al., 2012). In general, King et al. reported that girls experience more chronic pain than boys and that the experience of pain increases with age, into adolescence. They emphasized that more research into the correlates of chronic pain in boys and girls will be important. In their recent review, King et al. (2011) divided types of pain into major illnesses, such as pediatric headache, musculoskeletal pain, back pain, and abdominal pain to name a few. King et al. also assessed the occurrence of pain across several studies. Rates of pain varied widely across type of medical condition. For instance, rates of headache pain, the most common pain, varied from 8 to 83 % across studies. In epidemiological studies, children who reported more than one type of pain showed varying patterns ranging from 4 to 49 %. Hermann and Blanchard (2002) reported that as many as one-third of children could "outgrow" their experiences of pain, but they cautioned that this figure was an estimate and more longitudinal (long-term) studies of childhood pain are needed to determine whether this is the case.

Genetic and Environmental Influences

Genetic influences on pain may vary widely, based on the type of chronic illness. However, a review of studies using twins to examine heritability of pain across different types of medical problems does indicate that genetics influence pain responses (e.g., Nielsen, Knudsen, & Steingrímsdóttir, 2012). Heritability may be greatest for headache pain or perceptions of widespread pain responses without clear causes or symptoms. After this, back and neck pain may be influenced by genetic factors. Child temperament, which has a genetic component, also interacts with the aforementioned factors to determine children's adjustment to chronic medical conditions, which includes their adjustment to pain and their quality of life (Harper et al., 2014). For example, Walco (2008) reviewed several studies and determined that children who experience high anxiety levels and are very sensitive in nature might be more likely to experience pain. However, early negative experiences with pain may actually influence a child's long-term negative reactions to pain, making children more predisposed to experience pain in later years. This might be indicative of strong environmental determination of children's pain responses.

Developmental, environmental, and genetic factors may influence children's responses to painful experiences (Walco, 2008). A child's response to pain depends on his or her age (phase in development), genetic predisposition to feel pain, and the contextual or environmental factors that shape a child's pain response. In terms of contextual or environmental influences, children can learn how to cope with pain from observing others' pain responses. They also learn their pain responses based on reinforcement for their pain behaviors. For instance, whether or not the child him- or herself is reinforced by others, like parents, for the way he or she copes with pain may predispose a child to react more strongly to painful experiences. In support of environmental factors determining pain, results of a study examining low back pain in children indicated that the greatest impact on pain responses in children were environmental influences (El-Metwally et al., 2008). Environmental influences include several factors: early learning based on previous pain experiences, observation of others' responses to pain, and reinforcement of pain responses by significant others, such as parents and nurses.

Assessment

Education in pain assessment and management has become essential in the health professions and is considered a specialty area (Fein et al., 2012). There are many measurement tools used to assess children's pain responses. Visual analog scales (using a number line or a line with a point for low and high pain), for example, allow children to rate their pain on a scale from low to high pain, and these types of scales have been found to be useful in determining children's perceptions of their pain experiences. Pain faces, where children circle the face representing their pain, also can provide a good estimate of children's views of their pain experiences. For pain "faces" scales, children typically view several line drawings depicting happy faces and faces depicting distress and circle one or select one face to convey the nature of their pain (McGrath, 1990). In a fairly recent study with children between the ages of 4 and 17 years who were experiencing acute pain, Tsze, von Baeyer, Bulloch, and Dayan (2013) examined children's reports of pain using an analog scale (with visual markers and a slider to move to show their pain level) and a faces pain scale for children to convey how their pain was influencing them. These researchers found both of the aforementioned measures were good indicators of children's pain reports. They concluded that both measures were helpful and useful, because children reported lower pain on these measures after receiving treatment with analgesics. Both measures were sensitive to change in reports of severe pain. These researchers did report that more research on the use of pain measures would be necessary for children ages 7 years and younger because the utility of the scales used in this study was relatively weaker for children in this younger age group. Behavior observations and parent interviews may be useful for recording pain experiences for very young children, and they have been found to be good indicators for older children as well.

Wong and Baker (1988) used several types of scales to assess children's pain. They found that children enjoyed using a faces scale to report their pain. This type of scale might be recommended for children between the ages of 8 and 11 or 12 years of age. Children ages 13 and older might benefit from using a visual analog scale that allows them to rate their pain severity; then, they can describe how their pain feels and where their pain "hurts." In addition, it is necessary to ask children what causes them pain, because different procedures may be painful for different children, as pain is an individualized experience. Wong and Baker (1988) recommended that when assessing pain, one needs to ask the child how he or she is feeling, and use behavioral observations to determine the severity and frequency of the child's pain. They also cautioned that children may not become accustomed to pain, and therefore it is important to re-assess their symptoms over time.

Connelly et al. (2012) used electronic diaries to record how children and their parents responded to their children's arthritis pain. For this study, nine children and parents completed daily assessments of pain and mood using handheld computers. Assessments were recorded three times each day for 2 weeks. Study results indicated that parents who were overprotective of their children tended to have children who were less engaged in activities and who reported experiencing more negative mood states. Distraction could help children to stop "over-focusing" on pain, which, in turn, could help children engage in more activities. There was an exception to note, however. If children were experiencing "very high" disease activity, which typically involves high pain, then distraction and involvement in activities did not always lead to an improved mood state. This could have indicated that children were engaging in activities but not enjoying them or feeling well because their disease was at a more severe level. When pain reaches higher levels, consultation with pediatricians and pain management teams can offer support for the child. Research examining what types of strategies work (or do not work) given a child's experience of his or her pain intensity and his or her age level will make contributions to existing literature.

Impact on Children

Pain has a significant impact on children's lives. Children who experience pain may limit their involvement in activities and reduce time spent with their friends and children their own age. They may feel that they cannot control their pain and that no matter what they do the pain will always be there. Eccleston et al. (2012) mentioned that the experience of chronic, recurrent pain can have negative effects that last into adulthood. Others have confirmed that children's pain memories can shape their reactions to pain for the rest of their lives (e.g., Noel, Chambers, McGrath, Klein, & Stewart, 2012a, 2012b). Negative emotions also impact how a child experiences pain. Although pain can cause one to feel sad and anxious, these same feelings can actually increase a child's experience of pain. Catastrophizing (thinking the worst will happen in terms of thinking the pain will increase until it is unbearable) or feeling very out of control over one's pain can heighten a child's pain experience (Sullivan et al., 2001; Thastum, Herlin, & Zachariae, 2005). Hence, feeling that there is no way to control pain, may be related to increased reports of pain, such that a child who feels he or she cannot control pain will experience greater pain levels. Helping a child to work on believing that pain can decrease and that positive thinking can be used to reduce pain—that is, working on self-efficacy for coping with pain, can have a positive impact on how a child copes with pain.

There are several other factors that may impact children's pain experience. For instance, feelings of extreme anxiety or fear related to having pain can also increase the impact of pain for children. Moreover, if children have negative expectations about medical procedures, perhaps due to negative previous experiences, this can increase their pain when they undergo medical procedures. This can cause them to tense up, which may increase pain and it also causes distress, which can heighten the experience of pain. For example, if a child has had a bad experience, such as with a painful needle stick that caused bruising, he or she may expect another needle stick to be painful, increasing the painful nature of the experience and his or her distress level. A child can have a role in causing a negative experience, if he or she expects a very negative outcome or engages in catastrophizing or very negative thinking about how pain will occur (e.g., Sullivan et al., 2001). Specifically, a child's tension and muscle tightness, which may be anxiety-related, may cause a needle stick to hurt more.

Memories of painful experiences can play a role in children's reactions to new or current pain experiences. Recall of high intensity pain and the negative nature of this experience may be related to children reporting more pain in new pain-inducing situations (Noel et al., 2012a). Having experienced pain the past can also be related to a child experiencing more anxiety when needing to undergo new procedures that can cause pain. Thus, anxiety, negative pain experiences, and high intensity pain can influence each other in a negative cycle, such that negative memories of pain can cause new anxiety, heightening pain when the child is undergoing new painful procedures (Noel et al., 2012a). Consequently, pain memories should be explored with the child as negative memories can impact the child's abilities to deal with pain experiences.

Pain Management

Not understanding coping strategies, such as relaxation and distraction, can also leave children with a lack of tools for helping them manage their pain (Koller & Goldman, 2012). Relaxation can include thinking happy thoughts or listening to relaxing music. Distraction can occur through play or thinking about different, happy events. Using relaxation and distraction have the potential to help a child relax, making it less painful to undergo some medical procedures. Another long-term pain management strategy may be to have a child engage in gentle, regular exercise. Over the long run, gentle exercise can release endorphins which are the brains natural analgesic for helping pain coping. Moreover, restricted activity can increase stiffness and soreness, thereby increasing the child's pain.

Children may be reinforced, however inadvertently, by their parents when they report pain, causing their pain symptoms to recur or broaden in scope. Parents who show less distress about their children's pain are likely to have children who are functioning at a higher level (Sieberg, William, & Simons, 2011). A health professional may instruct a parent to de-emphasize the attention he or she pays to a child's expressions of pain, in order to provide a gentle "ignoring" experience, while the parent is encouraging the child to get back into the swing of his or her daily activities. If parents are too overprotective or too responsive to their child's report of pain, such as by decreasing the responsibilities he or she could perform, then the child can over-report or over-emphasize pain. In turn, his or her functioning suffers. Of course, this is not always the case, but this type of situation has been reported in the pain literature (e.g., Logan, Simons, & Carpino, 2012). One strategy for children with long-term chronic pain is for a parent to encourage his or her child to "get back into life" and re-engage in activities and time spent with friends. Ignoring pain and encouraging activity can be tricky. This can be a delicate balance, as children's reports of pain can be under-emphasized. If this occurs, then children can be under-medicated and not get the medicine they need to relieve pain. Using observation and assessing a child's pain regularly over time can provide data for health educators and parents to inform their decisions about responding to a child's reports of pain.

In their review of management of acute pain in children, Samuel, Steiner, and Shavit (2014) noted that children with injuries may not receive appropriate levels of analgesia to treat their pain symptoms, indicating that they are under-medicated in terms of pain treatment. They noted several possible reasons for this lack of treatment, including potential exaggerated fears of medication effects for children (i.e., worrying that the child could become addicted to pain medications) or fears of adverse events related to medication for children. They concluded that more studies with children, especially very young children, to understand the management of acute pain, are needed.

Parents are role models for their child. If a parent thinks the worst will happen, because the child is in pain, the child can come to believe this assumption. Children can learn a pain response from others who have pain, and thus, if parents experience pain themselves, they need to consider role-modeling positive coping, using distraction, positive thinking, and relaxation, to help them cope with their pain. If parents hold a catastrophizing attitude, believing the worst will occur or that pain is very limiting, the child can model this attitude. In fact, Logan et al. (2012) reported that parents who were overly sympathetic to the child's report of pain may have influenced the child's tendency to avoid going to school. Parents who are overly sympathetic to their child or have a negative view of outcomes may be more likely to think that teachers' responses to the child's pain are not as sympathetic as they could be.

It is important to mention that parents may be the key champions in helping their child overcome pain or have a positive attitude toward a painful experience. In fact, in a study measuring a pain management program for children with cancer, McCarthy et al. (2013) found that parents were likely to use distraction, humor, or help their child with deep breathing to assist their child in coping with pain. Their primary or number one strategy was distraction, and comforting the child by holding him or her was a close second, in terms of helping the child through a painful

Table 4.1 Pain management strategies for children

Name of pain channel	Explanation and strategies
Positive thoughts	Helping the child think of positive things to say to him or herself can help the child fight his or her pain
	Teach the child to "Think away your pain. Your brain understands the pain message. If you think you can beat your pain you can make it less! Having a positive attitude can really help you make your pain lower. What kinds of things can help you have a positive attitude and be happy? Let's think about how you can do something that makes you happy every day"
Getting help from other people	Other people like teachers can help a child when he or she has a pain flare. Children need to ask others for help ("Talking to an adult to tell them you need a break to help your pain go lower is a good pain strategy."). Health educators should teach others (teachers, coaches, even friends) how to help a child cope with pain
Doing something fun	Doing something fun, like playing a game to help as a distraction strategy. Make sure that the activity is something the child considers fun, as strategies will vary for different children
	Teach children to use their imaginations to do something fun in their minds or brain, like thinking of a favorite activity or going to the beach. This type of distraction is "imagery." Make sure that the child thinks about all the details of the situation to make the image as vivid as possible (e.g., sights, sounds, smells). Another type of imagery for children that also allows children to challenge their pain is to have them imagine their own special superhero who is challenging their pain and beating it!
Relaxation	The relaxation response is different from the uptight and ramped up nature of the pain response in many children. Have children do something relaxing like listen to music or watch television. Warm compresses can also help children relax. Finally, some children can do a modified version of muscle relaxation where they tense and relax their fists or feet (if these areas are not in pain) to try to relax their bodies
Gentle movement	Moving, typically through gentle exercise (check each child's tolerance level) may help the child to reduce his or her pain. Have the child start with low activity or movement and go slow. Always make sure that a movement strategy is acceptable to the child's doctor

experience. Parents were present more than 95 % of the time for children ages 8 and younger who were coping with painful events. Hence, the primary agent for teaching a child to manage pain may be parents, and teaching parents pain management strategies so that they can practice them with their child may be a very successful experience for the parent and child.

Table 4.1 presents several strategies, such as getting support from others, distraction, imagery, and relaxation, that may help children manage their pain.

The strategies reviewed in Table 4.1 provide some guidelines for health professionals interested in using psychosocial pain management strategies with children. The strategies presented in this table are primarily behavioral. However, imagery is a cognitive strategy. It is important to consider training in other specialty areas to provide therapy for children experiencing pain. Some of these areas include music and art therapy as well as participating in training in how to use hypnosis, biofeedback, or message.

Hypnosis involves helping the child to attain an inner state of intense concentration and focused attention (Kohen & Kaiser, 2014). Experts have proposed that the state of focused attention discovered in hypnotic states in children can be induced by imagery, intensely focusing on thoughts or objects, or intensely focusing on breathing (Kohen & Kaiser, 2014). Children may be especially responsive to statements that suggest their pain will be reduced and that they will be more relaxed when hypnosis is used, because children may be more responsive to suggestion when they are in a hypnotic state. The author of this chapter is not an expert on the use of hypnosis and a detailed explanation of how to use hypnosis or hypnotic induction with children is beyond the scope of this chapter. Those interested in gaining a greater understanding of hypnosis are guided to the National Pediatric Hypnosis Training Institute (http://www.nphti.net/) and to review books on the subject, such as one entitled, "Therapeutic Hypnosis with Children and Adolescents" by Sugarman and Wester (2013).

Biofeedback is another intervention (it is not reviewed in Table 4.1) that can be used to manage children's pain. When biofeedback is used to manage a child's pain, he or she is connected to a monitoring device that shows the child's pulse, respiration rate, or skin temperature. The child then can learn through visual feedback and by paying attention to his or her body, in order to learn which body states are associated with lower arousal and stress. Through monitoring one's bodily states and practicing relaxation or diaphragmatic breathing, the child can learn to control a stressful physiological reaction. Children can learn to lower their heart rates, respiration rates, and body temperatures, decreasing the pain response. This type of training allows the child to train his or her autonomic nervous system so that he or she will be more relaxed, reducing the pain response. The autonomic nervous system works without conscious effort and regulates automatic body processes, like breathing. The notion is that if physiological reactivity is controlled when the child relaxes or reduces physiological reactivity, then the child's pain response can be reduced. Repeated training sessions are needed for the child to learn a more relaxed physiological response. It is recommended that clinicians and health educators receive special training and practice under supervision to learn how to use this technique effectively. Research has shown that biofeedback has been effective in reducing pain related to pediatric headache, especially migraines (Hermann & Blanchard, 2002), and in reducing abdominal pain in children with Irritable Bowel Syndrome and functional abdominal pain (Stern, Guiles, & Gevirtz, 2014). Biofeedback can be used with other pain management techniques such as muscle relaxation or breathing as a combination treatment to combat children's pain (Hermann & Blanchard, 2002).

Gentle massage (touch) may be another tool to help a child combat pain. Field (1996) has documented the benefits of massage for children with chronic medical conditions such as asthma, diabetes, and burns. For children with burn injuries, she found that massage was related to decreased reports of pain. Field also discovered lower pain reports for adults with fibromyalgia who participated in message. Typically, gentle touch was used for a period of 30 min or less. Field speculated that decreases in stress levels could be related to the positive impact of message. Special training and supervision would be recommended for those learning this type of intervention.

It is essential to consider the child's general orientation to gaining information and coping with pain, when helping the child learn to manage pain. If the child is an information seeker, and benefits from learning about procedures and how to manage pain, then providing him or her with medical information about his or her condition or medical procedures may be helpful. Demonstrating how a medical procedure will work and explaining how it occurs can actually be soothing for a child who is an information-seeker. Some children may even benefit from assisting with the procedure, such as telling the doctor or nurse "when" to do a needle stick. On the other hand, if a child is a "distractor" by nature, then the child might benefit from distracting him or herself by having fun (engaging in a fun activity), using imagery (thinking of a favorite activity), or using relaxation (breathing or blowing bubbles). It is most likely that a combination of strategies will work for children and it may be that different strategies will work in different situations and at different times.

Parental support and comfort are excellent pain management strategies for most children. Many children look to their parents for comfort and to provide distraction. Others observe their parents who are "models" showing the child how to cope with pain. Adults must monitor how their child is reacting to them as a "support" in managing pain, because as support-persons they can help or harm their child's pain management efforts. As mentioned, if adults in the home pay a great deal of attention to children's pain reports, then the children's reports of their pain symptoms can potentially increase and the children may experience decreased levels of social functioning and involvement in their daily lives (Peterson & Palermo, 2004; Walker, Claar, & Garber, 2002). Therefore, it is recommended that parents acknowledge children's pain and help them treat it. On the other hand, it is also necessary for parents to make sure that they do not overprotect their child when he or she reports pain. They should also make sure that to the extent possible, their child engages in daily activities and socializes. Withdrawing from social and daily experiences can cause depression and anxiety in children and heighten the nature of pain experiences. Instead parents should foster active coping with pain, assisting in teaching their child positive pain coping strategies such as relaxation and encouraging them to carry on with daily functioning (Connelly et al., 2012). Health educators need to gather information on a case by case basis as there may be variations in parent responses and variations in child needs when making recommendations about pain management. After a comprehensive literature review, Eccleston et al. (2012) emphasized that psychological and behavioral treatments for pain should be tailored to both the child and family's needs.

Medications

The administration of medication to manage pain is complex and a detailed description is beyond the scope of this chapter. In many children's hospitals, a pain management team, consisting of physicians, nurses, and other health professionals, may specialize in caring for children's pain. This team may make recommendations for their pediatricians to manage their pain after they leave the hospital. Pain teams may develop pre-measured doses of pain medications and children can administer pain medicine through pushing a button which delivers a small dose of pain medication through intravenous lines. The amount of drug available to the child is measured so that the child has access to the "correct" amount of the medication (the dose that the child is to have over a specific time interval); however, the child can administer the medication in small doses over a certain time period. Having control of the administration of medication can help a child feel that he or she has some control over the pain that he or she is experiencing.

Berde and Sethna (2002) provided guidelines for the use of analgesics in treating children's pain. They discussed the use of aspirin, acetaminophen, or nonsteroidal anti-inflammatory drugs (NSAIDS), such as ibuprofen and naproxen, in children. They mentioned that opioids have been used in the treatment of pain related to cancer and sickle cell disease for children. Opioids have also been used to treat postoperative pain. Research has not indicated that children become addicted to these medications. Fein et al. (2012) recommended that physicians in the emergency room consider administration of an analgesic if a child's level of pain is greater than three on a rating scale from 0 to 10. Contraindications for administration of an analgesic are if the child is allergic to a pain medication. Ibuprofen can be used, unless the child has an allergy to aspirin, has an upcoming surgery, or has a bleeding disorder or renal disease. Acetaminophen was another choice for pain relief as well as oral oxycodone. Topical anesthetics, such as EMLA, could be used to control pain related to IV catheter placement and other minor procedures. EMLA is a topical anesthetic or cream that children can rub on an external area of skin where there might be a needle stick and it will numb this area. Medical professionals should follow guidelines and decision trees for administration of medications with children, in order to consider the many possibilities and contraindications for using pain medications with children.

Psychosocial Factors Related to Pain and Emotional Functioning

Children who experience significant chronic pain are likely to miss school, withdraw from friends and social activities, and they are at risk for internalizing problems, such as depression and/or anxiety (McGrath, 1990; Weiss et al., 2013). Family relationships can be strained as parents experience anxiety when their child is in pain.

Children may view events in their lives in a negative light when they are in pain. King et al. (2011) found various relationships among psychosocial factors and different medical conditions which typically involve pain. For example, children residing in low-income families were more likely to report headache pain. Children with recurrent abdominal pain were often likely to experience anxiety and/or depression. Similarly, children reporting back pain also could be experiencing anxiety and/or depression. After reviewing studies assessing "general" reports of pain, King et al. discovered that children reporting pain experienced a lower quality of life than for children who did not report experiencing chronic pain. Thus, psychosocial factors associated with pain vary by type of medical condition, but it is important to consider these factors when assessing chronic pain for children with different types of medical conditions.

In an earlier review article, Lavigne, Schulein, and Hahn (1986) reported that children who are likely to experience pain may be more anxious and insecure; they could tend to be "emotionally reactive." They may be worriers and perfectionists in that they are overachievers, who are overly conscientious. However, this typology or "pain type" is not supported by all studies. Indeed, Lavigne et al. noted that there are many factors that may determine a child's pain response, including family history of pain and how parents respond to a child's reports of pain. Pain typology appears more complex than just a child personality type. For example, Harper et al. (2014) found children who had a bounce back, positive, or resilient attitude were better able to cope with having cancer, which is a disease accompanied by many painful procedures. It may be that resilient children, with easy-going temperaments, are better able to cope with pain. This is encouraging because teaching children how to become more positive is a skill that can be learned and mastered.

Children who are experiencing pain may experience higher levels of depression, irrespective of the physically limiting nature of their pain experience (Kashikar-Zuck, Goldschneider, Power, Vaught, & Hershey, 2001). Kashikar-Zuck and her colleagues examined the impact of chronic pain in 73 children with chronic pain that were followed for 1 year at a pediatric outpatient clinic. They reported that children with chronic pain experience "significant difficulties in psychosocial functioning" (p. 346). Children experience disruption in school, either missing school or having to be home-schooled. Most of the patients they surveyed showed mild to moderate levels of depression, which could have been either an outgrowth of or a precursor to their pain experience. It was of concern that about 15 % of the sample reported significant levels of depression, which indicated a need for long-term psychological treatment.

In addition, children may need psychological support to reduce isolation and feelings of depression related to having chronic pain. Kashikar-Zuck et al. (2001) noted that a pattern of negative thinking and believing the worst would happen could be related to experiencing higher levels of pain. Teaching children to interrupt negative thinking cycles and speak more positively to themselves (i.e., engage in more positive self-talk) may be a key skill to help children change negative thinking that may amplify their pain experience.

Lacking sleep can be a factor in children's pain experience (Chambers, Corkum, & Rusak, 2008). Specifically, children who have difficulty sleeping may report higher levels of pain. In a study with children who had arthritis, Bromberg, Gil, and Schanberg (2012) found that poor sleep quality was related to higher reports of pain for children with arthritis. Positive mood states could mitigate or change this relationship, such that when children were feeling positively the relationship between poor sleep and pain was not as strong. Interestingly, children's experience of pain did not predict their sleep quality the next evening. This meant that although poor sleep was related to experiencing pain the next day, the reverse was not the case in this study (i.e., pain during the day did not predict poor sleep quality at night).

Interventions

Palermo and her colleagues examined research reviewing the impact of psychological therapies to help children combat pain (Palermo, Eccleston, Lewandowski, Williams, & Morley, 2010). The studies considered in the review by Palermo and her colleagues were randomized controlled trails. In these types of studies, children have a random chance of being assigned to a treatment or a wait-list control group. The wait-list control group usually receives treatment right after or a short time after the treatment group has received the treatment. If the treatment group is faring better in terms of functioning and quality of life compared to the control group, then the authors may conclude that the treatment is having a positive impact. Palermo et al. (2010) reported that psychological treatment had a positive influence on children's psychological functioning and reduced the "disability" they experienced related to their pain. In terms of the treatments, many seemed to be between 8 and 10 sessions, occurring weekly or more frequently (such as two times a week). Progress was measured using pain diaries, where children recorded their pain, and other measures assessing emotional functioning, quality of life, etc. Treatments varied and included relaxation, biofeedback, imagery, and other cognitive-behavioral treatments, similar in nature to those described in Table 4.1.

Multicomponent Interventions. Many pain interventions for children involve more than one treatment and are thus called multicomponent treatment interventions. For instance, multicomponent treatment interventions may involve relaxation, biofeedback, distraction, and pain medications. A multicomponent intervention may also involve pain medication and cognitive therapy to help children manage painful thoughts, relax, and control negative or catastrophic thinking. Another type of multicomponent intervention might be a program including gentle stretching and exercise, medication and psychological interventions (e.g., positive coping and positive imagery [thinking positive and relaxing thoughts]) to help a child control pain.

Schiff, Holtz, Peterson, and Rakusan (2001) assessed the influence of a multiple component intervention to reduce pain and distress for children with HIV. Participants in their intervention were between 4 and 12 years of age and had HIV. The children were in relatively good health. These researchers conducted a single group design. Thus, there was not a control group, where children in the group were on a waiting list and did not participate in the intervention. They assessed children's functioning and adjustment over time, using repeated measurements. The pain management intervention focused on using EMLA cream to numb the skin and using relaxation (breathing) to help children with venipunctures. Children also received knowledge about what was going to happen and viewed a demonstration of procedures using a doll. Observers noted the children's pain responses during procedures and children completed a pain scale with faces and a visual analog scale to provide data about their pain. Parents completed a measure examining their anxiety. Results indicated that the intervention was successful in reducing child report of pain and parent anxiety. An observer noted less behavioral distress during venipunctures (Schiff et al., 2001). With multicomponent treatment studies, such as this one, it is not possible to tell whether one aspect of the treatment was the effective component (above and beyond the impact of the other components), such that this one component was behind the positive change. However, in general, results were positive, and provide further support for the positive impact of psychological interventions to improve children's pain.

Weiss et al. (2013) described a rehabilitation program to assist children and adolescents manage their pain. This program had many interventions and thus could be considered a multicomponent intervention. Participants were between 11 and 18 years of age. Children participated in treatment that allowed them to learn critical pain management strategies such as distraction, positive self-talk, relaxation, and biofeedback. Children also could participate in psychotherapy if they were experiencing other psychological problems, such as anxiety or depression. Alleviating internalizing symptoms can be a component of pain management. Weiss et al. described family therapy and teaching parents to stop reinforcing child report and experience of pain symptoms as critical components of treatment. They recommended light exercise as a key treatment for children's pain. In their rehabilitation program, children also participated in recreation and play therapy. Recreation can help children move and have fun, both key treatments for pain. Play therapy can help children work through emotions and improve their acceptance of their chronic medical condition, and this too can be an important pain management strategy. In the comprehensive program described by Weiss et al., children also participated in occupational and physical therapy, which can "rehab" muscles that have atrophied due to not being used. Atrophy can occur when muscles are not used, and then they become weak and it can hurt when one begins to use them again. Weiss et al. found that when children were more able to accept their pain, feelings of depression decreased and child functioning increased. Weiss et al.'s results suggested acceptance could be a contributing factor to a positive attitude, although other factors could contribute to depression, child thoughts about pain, and child functioning. Children with chronic pain may experience depression and anxiety as well as have problems with social functioning and achievement at school (Weiss et al., 2013).

Roles for Health Educators

There are many roles for health educators to assist children in improving their pain coping. For instance, they can administer measures and track children's pain experiences using surveys and observations for the medical team or to provide information for pediatricians treating the child. They can educate parents and health professionals about the fact that young children may be under-medicated and that there is a myth that children will become addicted to pain medications. They can teach parents and health professionals about how to model appropriate pain coping responses and ways to lessen inadvertent reinforcement of the pain response by providing too much attention and sympathy for the child's pain reactions. Parents may inadvertently influence children's pain responses, through paying too much attention to children's reports of pain or allowing children to miss too many activities. When parents inadvertently reinforce children's pain responses, then reports of pain can increase. Thus, it is vital for health educators to teach parents coping strategies so that they can work with children to actively deal with their pain and return to their daily routines.

Health educators can teach children and their caregivers about the pain management strategies detailed in Table 4.1 and throughout this chapter. Those educators with expertise in helping children cope with internalizing symptoms, especially depression, such as licensed counselors and psychologists can provide treatment for depression and anxiety for children. Many children will benefit from engaging in positive self-statements (e.g., I can make my pain less") to help them distract themselves when they are in pain. Developing multicomponent interventions for children and finding a role on pain management teams in hospital settings may be other opportunities for health educators.

Case Study

Brandon is an 8-year-old boy, who is described as a very sensitive child. He is likely to experience migraine headaches, especially when he is stressed at school. Brandon is "just like his mother" who also experiences stress-related headache pain. Brandon presented at the headache clinic and the attending physician (this is the physician who leads the clinic team) believed that a consultation with a health educator might help Brandon and his mother develop some cognitive-behavioral strategies to help him to manage his pain. Brandon has frequent headaches, primarily at school. His mother noted that the headaches occur at school, "…Eighty percent of the time and at home about 20 % of the time." She mentioned that Brandon can become tired of being at school, especially in the afternoons when he has not eaten well at lunch. The headaches begin with him "seeing a light on his right side." He often needs to go to a dark room to feel better. Sometimes a nap will help him to sleep away his migraine. Brandon's mother referred him to see a health educator working in the schools. She asked if the health educator could talk with her son to help him develop strategies to deal with headache pain so that he could remain in school and miss fewer afternoons due to having migraines.

The health educator first met with Brandon's mother to take notes and learn of relevant background information. Brandon's history was relatively unremarkable with a normal birth history and normal development as a youngster. Despite his school absences, his grades were good and he had several good friends at school as well as in his neighborhood. His presenting problem (the problem that needed to improve) was contained to migraines. His pediatrician had already referred him to a pediatric neurologist in private practice. The pediatric neurologist had suggested seeking counseling as an adjunctive treatment to medication management.

The health educator asked Brandon's mother about how she handled Brandon's pain. She reported that she "stopped everything" when he complained of pain and immediately told him to rest. She often provided him with cookies and milk, a favorite treat, when he had to cope with migraine pain. She spent on-on-one time with him, which was a rarity, because she was a working mother with a fairly demanding job. She did note that thinking of fun things appeared to be a favorite strategy of Brandon's for coping with things that were hard for him, and that this strategy seemed to work well before his migraine pain became too intense.

The health educator held a session with Brandon's mother to review her behavior and show her how she might be reinforcing Brandon's pain reports and pain behaviors. Brandon's mother agreed to help him rest when he had a migraine; however, she agreed to stop providing him with treats and intensive sympathy when he reported migraine pain. Instead, she agreed to save treats for accomplishments and special occasions. She also agreed to spend special time, 10–15 min per day, with Brandon. This special time would always "be there" for Brandon and she would try not to provide him with lots of attention and private time with her when he complained of pain.

The health educator also met with Brandon at school. Brandon described his headaches as beginning with, "a little pain on top of my eyebrows." Then, if he saw a light on his right, he might get more intense pain that could become a migraine headache. Brandon did not think he had any strategies to cope with his pain. The health educator subsequently reviewed deep, diaphragmatic breathing with Brandon and she reviewed how to use imagery in terms of thinking about happy and relaxing thoughts to help Brandon cope with pain. Brandon agreed to practice his strategies nightly with his mother. His imagery or positive memory strategy was to imagine the Incredible Hulk using his hammer and strength to hit a pain block. Brandon pictured his migraine pain as a cement block of pain weighing down his head. The Hulk would break it up so it would not weigh down his head. This Hulk story is a good example of an individual's particular imagery strategy, as many might see the Hulk's actions as ones that might cause pain; however, Brandon saw the Hulk as a pain hero and his actions had a calming and relaxing impact for this child.

Brandon was instructed to use his breathing and imagery when he first felt tension above his eyebrows. He practiced his strategies three times a week. He agreed to use his strategies as soon as possible if he felt pain. Brandon was able to use the strategies early in his pain cycle. Therefore, he had fewer migraines and the migraines he did experience had lessened in intensity. His mother also noted that her relationship with her son was going well and seemed based more on positive time spent together rather than time spent focusing on his migraines. The health educator agreed to check in with Brandon on a monthly basis to ensure his headaches were not interfering with his school progress and daily functioning. The health educator also received a release of information form from Brandon's mother so that she could share information with the child's pediatric neurologist, teacher, school nurse, and pediatrician, which helped disseminate information about treatment. The resolution of this case was successful. It is noteworthy that this is a best case scenario, and often parents and children may not be as quick to respond to interventions or practice psychosocial strategies that can lessen pain experiences.

Summary

In this chapter we learned that a significant number of children experience pain and need treatment for their pain. In addition, we learned about how to explain how pain works in the body to children. Pain is subjective in nature and thus taking an individualized approach in assessing children's pain is important. Ideas for assessing children's pain experiences, such as through the use of scales with faces or visual analog scales were described. Coping strategies may include relaxation, imagery, distraction, and muscle relaxation. Other strategies, which may take a lot of special training to implement, include massage, hypnosis, and biofeedback training. Multicomponent interventions or treatment packages, consisting of several interventions, often are used to treat children's pain. These interventions have been successful, but when treatment packages are used it is not possible to determine which of the interventions in the package had the most advantageous impact on lessening children's pain. On the other hand, cognitive-behavioral strategies, such as positive imagery and relaxation techniques, such as breathing, can have a positive impact on children's pain perceptions. Health educators can play a key role in educating children and parents about how pain works and about strategies to facilitate pain management. Interventions to reduce children's pain experience need to be evaluated, in order to continue to advance knowledge in the field.

Exercises/Questions

1. Pain is subjective in nature. Briefly explain what is meant by this statement.
2. Provide a developmentally appropriate explanation of how pain messages work in the body for an elementary school-age child.
3. Parents or caregivers can reinforce pain and change a child's pain experience. Please provide a description of how a parent could increase a child's pain response.
4. Describe ideas for relaxation and imagery strategies to help children cope with pain.

5. If you were a pain management specialist in a pain clinic, how would you recommend working with depression in children experiencing pain? What would be some interventions you would suggest to treat both symptoms of depression and pain in children with both conditions?
6. In the case study, Brandon's pain improved with interventions. How would you recommend assessing Brandon's perceptions of his pain if you were collecting information on his responses to pain interventions?

Key Concepts

Nociception
Referred pain
Causalgia pain
Nociceptive processing
Reinforcement of a child's pain responses
Catastrophizing attitude
Imagery
Visual analog scale
Hypnosis
Biofeedback
NSAIDS
EMLA
Resilient attitude
Multicomponent interventions

References

Berde, C. B., & Sethna, N. F. (2002). Analgesics for the treatment of pain in children. *New England Journal of Medicine, 347*(14), 1094–1103.

Bromberg, M. H., Gil, K. M., & Schanberg, L. E. (2012). Daily sleep quality and mood as predictors of pain in children with juvenile polyarticular arthritis. *Health Psychology, 31*(2), 202–209. doi:10.1037/a0025075.

Bromberg, M. H., Schechter, N. L., Nurko, S., Zempsky, W. T., & Schanberg, L. E. (2014). Persistent pain in chronically ill children without detectable disease activity. *Pain Management, 4*(3), 211–219. doi:10.2217/pmt.14.6.

Chambers, C., Corkum, P. V., & Rusak, B. (2008). Commentary: The importance of sleep in pediatric chronic pain—A wakeup call for pediatric psychologists. *Journal of Pediatric Psychology, 33*, 339–348.

Connelly, M., Bromberg, M. H., Anthony, K. K., Gil, K. M., Franks, L., & Schanberg, L. E. (2012). Emotion regulation predicts pain and functioning in children with juvenile idiopathic arthritis: An electronic diary study. *Journal of Pediatric Psychology, 37*(1), 43–52.

Eccleston, C., Palermo, T. M., de C Williams, A. C., Lewandowski, A., Morley, S., Fisher, E., & Law, E. (2012). Psychological therapies for the management of chronic and recurrent pain in children and adolescents. *The Cochrane Database of Systematic Reviews, 12*, CD003968. doi:10.1002/14651858.CD003968.pub3.

El-Metwally, A., Mikkelsson, M., Ståhl, M., Macfarlane, G. J., Jones, G. T., Pulkkinen, L., … Kaprio, J. (2008). Genetic and environmental influences on non-specific low back pain in children: A twin study. *European Spine Journal, 17*(4), 502–508.

Fein, J. A., Zempsky, W. T., Cravero, J., & The Committee on Pediatric Emergency Medicine and Section on Anesthesiology and Pain Medicine. (2012). Relief of pain and anxiety in pediatric patients in emergency medical systems. *Pediatrics, 130*(5), e1391–e1405. doi:10.1542/peds.2012-2536.

Field, T. M. (1996). Touch therapies for pain management and stress reduction. In R. J. Resnick & R. H. Rozensky (Eds.), *Health psychology through the life span: Practice and research opportunities* (pp. 313–321). Washington, DC: American Psychological Association.

Harper, F. W., Goodlett, B. D., Trentacosta, C. J., Albrecht, T. L., Taub, J. W., Phipps, S., & Penner, L. A. (2014). Temperament, personality, and quality of life in pediatric cancer patients. *Journal of Pediatric Psychology, 39*(4), 459–468.

Hermann, C., & Blanchard, E. B. (2002). Biofeedback in the treatment of headache and other childhood pain. *Applied Psychophysiology and Biofeedback, 27*(2), 143–162.

Kashikar-Zuck, S., Goldschneider, K. R., Power, S. W., Vaught, M. H., & Hershey, A. D. (2001). Depression and functional disability in chronic pediatric pain. *Clinical Journal of Pain, 17*, 341–349.

King, S., Chambers, C. T., Huguet, A., MacNevin, R. C., McGrath, P. J., Parker, L., & MacDonald, A. J. (2011). The epidemiology of chronic pain in children and adolescents revisited: A systematic review. *Pain, 152*(12), 2729–2738. doi:10.1016/j.pain.2011.07.016.

Kohen, D. P., & Kaiser, P. (2014). Clinical hypnosis with children and adolescents—What? Why? How?: Origins, applications, and efficacy. *Children, 1*(2), 74–98. doi:10.3390/children1020074.

Koller, D., & Goldman, R. D. (2012). Distraction techniques for children undergoing procedures: A critical review of pediatric research. *Journal of Pediatric Nursing, 27*(6), 652–681.

Lavigne, J. V., Schulein, M. J., & Hahn, Y. S. (1986). Psychological aspects of painful medical conditions in children. II. Personality factors, family characteristics and treatment. *Pain, 27*, 147–169.

Logan, D. E., Simons, L. E., & Carpino, E. A. (2012). Too sick for school? Parent influences on school functioning among children with chronic pain. *Pain, 153*, 437–443. doi:10.1016/j.pain.2011.11.004.

McCarthy, M., Glick, R., Green, J., Plummer, K., Peters, K., Johnsey, L., & DeLuca, C. (2013). Comfort First: An evaluation of a procedural pain management programme for children with cancer. *Psycho-Oncology, 22*, 775–782. doi:10.1002/pon.3061.

McGrath, P. A. (1990). *Pain in children: Nature, assessment, and treatment*. New York, NY: Guilford.

Melzak, R., & Wall, P. D. (1965). Pain mechanisms: A new theory. *Science, 150*, 971–979.

National Institute of Neurological Disorders and Stroke (NINDS). (2015). Pain: Hope through research. Retrieved December 9, 2015, from http://www.ninds.nih.gov/disorders/chronic_pain/detail_chronic_pain.htm.

Nielsen, C. S., Knudsen, G. P., & Steingrímsdóttir, Ó. A. (2012). Twin studies of pain. *Clinical Genetics, 82*(4), 331–340.

Noel, M., Chambers, C. T., McGrath, P. J., Klein, R. M., & Stewart, S. H. (2012a). The influence of children's pain memories on subsequent pain experience. *Pain, 153*(8), 1563–1572.

Noel, M., Chambers, C. T., McGrath, P. J., Klein, R. M., & Stewart, S. H. (2012b). The role of state anxiety in children's memories for pain. *Journal of Pediatric Psychology, 37*(5), 567–579. doi:10.093/jpepsy/jss006.

Palermo, T. M., Eccleston, C., Lewandowski, A. S., Williams, A. C., & Morley, S. (2010). Randomized controlled trials of psychological therapies for management of chronic pain in children and adolescents: An updated meta-analytic review. *Pain, 148*, 387–397. doi:10.1016/j.pain.2009.10.004.

Peterson, C., & Palermo, T. (2004). Parental reinforcement of recurrent pain: The moderating impact of child depression and anxiety on functional disability. *Journal of Pediatric Psychology, 29*, 331–341.

Samuel, N., Steiner, I. P., & Shavit, I. (2014). Prehospital pain management of injured children: A systematic review of current evidence. *American Journal of Emergency Medicine, 33*(3), 451–454. doi:10.1016/j.ajem.2014.12.012.

Schiff, W. B., Holtz, K. D., Peterson, N., & Rakusan, T. (2001). Effect of an intervention to reduce procedural pain and distress for children with HIV infection. *Journal of Pediatric Psychology, 26*(7), 417–427.

Sieberg, C. B., William, S., & Simons, L. E. (2011). Do parent protective responses mediate the relation between parent distress and child functional disability among children with chronic pain? *Journal of Pediatric Psychology, 36*(9), 1043–1051. doi:10.1093/jpepsy/jsr043.

Stern, M. J., Guiles, R. A. F., & Gevirtz, R. (2014). HRV biofeedback for pediatric irritable bowel syndrome and functional abdominal pain: A clinical replication series. *Applied Psychophysiology and Biofeedback, 39*, 287–291. doi:10.1007/s10484-014-9261-x.

Sugarman, L. I., & Wester, W. C. (Eds.). (2013). *Therapeutic hypnosis with children and adolescents.* Bancyfelin Carmarthen, England: Crown House Publishing.

Sullivan, M. J., Thorn, B., Haythornthwaite, J. A., Keefe, F., Martin, M., Bradley, L. A., & Lefebvre, J. C. (2001). Theoretical perspectives on the relation between catastrophizing and pain. *Clinical Journal of Pain, 17*(1), 52–64.

Thastum, M., Herlin, T., & Zachariae, R. (2005). Relationship of pain-coping strategies and pain-specific beliefs to pain experience in children with juvenile idiopathic arthritis. *Arthritis Care and Research, 53*(2), 178–184.

Tsze, D. S., von Baeyer, C. L., Bulloch, B., & Dayan, P. S. (2013). Validation of self-report pain scales in children. *Pediatrics, 132*, e971–e979. doi:10.1542/peds2013-1509.

Walco, G. A. (2008). Needle pain in children: Contextual factors. *Pediatrics, 122*(Supplement 3), S125–S129. doi:10.1542/peds.2008-1055d.

Walker, L., Claar, R., & Garber, J. (2002). Social consequences of children's pain: When do they encourage symptom maintenance? *Journal of Pediatric Psychology, 27*, 689–698.

Weiss, K. E., Hahn, A., Wallace, D. P., Biggs, B., Bruce, B. K., & Harrison, T. E. (2013). Acceptance of pain: Associations with depression, catastrophizing, and functional disability among children and adolescents in an interdisciplinary chronic pain rehabilitation program. *Journal of Pediatric Psychology, 38*(7), 756–765. doi:10.1093/jpepsy/jst028.

Wong, D. L., & Baker, C. M. (1988). Pain in children: Comparison of assessment scales. *Pediatric Nursing, 14*(1), 9–17.

Chapter 5
Cancer

Diagnosis

The American Cancer Society is a key source for information on cancer in children. Cancers are caused by abnormal cell growth in the body that is excessive. The cancer cells can grow and form a tumor or invade other tissues in the body. The cancer cells have damaged DNA that does not repair or die. The abnormal cells, which the body does not need, keep replicating. The new cells have the same abnormal DNA (http://www.cancer.org/cancer/braincnstumorsinchildren/detailedguide/brain-and-spinal-cord-tumors-in-children-what-is-cancer; downloaded on October 4, 2015).

Cancer is often difficult to detect. Many symptoms may signal childhood cancer. These may include an unusual mass or swelling, paleness, fatigue, easy bruising, prolonged fever, headaches (with vomiting), and weight loss (Ward, DeSantis, Robbins, Kohler, & Jemal, 2014). Other symptoms may include: limping, vision changes, and fever or illness that does not go away (http://www.cancer.org/cancer/cancerinchildren/detailedguide/cancer-in-children-finding-childhood-cancers-early; downloaded on October 4, 2015). Leukemias, which are cancers of the bone marrow and blood, are the most common types of childhood cancers (http://www.cancer.org/cancer/cancerinchildren/detailedguide/cancer-in-children-types-of--childhood-cancers; downloaded October 4, 2015).

Acute Lymphoblastic Leukemia (ALL) is the most common type of cancer in young children. There are 3,000 children in the United States with ALL each year (https://www.stjude.org/disease/acute-lymphoblastic-leukemia-all.html, downloaded October 4, 2015). Symptoms of ALL include easy bruising, pain, tiredness, flat red spots on the skin which are blood under the skin (petechiae), pain in bones and joints, experiencing frequent infections, and possible lumps in the neck, stomach, or groin areas. ALL is characterized by immature white blood cells in the bone marrow and these blood cells are unable to fight infections. In addition, white blood cells (lymphocytes) can build up in the liver, lymph nodes, and spleen. Treatments include chemotherapy, radiation, and stem cell transplant (the patient receives

© Springer International Publishing Switzerland 2016
L. Nabors, *Medical and Mental Health During Childhood*, Springer
Series on Child and Family Studies, DOI 10.1007/978-3-319-31117-3_5

healthy blood cells from a donor). Treatment of ALL includes prolonged chemo-therapy and in some cases bone marrow transplantation. When ALL is in remission, children are at risk for cognitive and neurological impairment, growth deficiencies, and risks for other types of cancers. ALL peaks in children between the ages of 2 and 5 years (Spector, Pankratz, & Marcotte, 2015). In a recent study, experts from the Children's Oncology Group reported that greater than 90 % of children with ALL would be cured, and that many would receive intensive treatment regimens lasting for 2–3 years (Myers et al., 2014).

Brain tumors and cancers of the central nervous system are the next most common types of cancers in children (Dolecek, Propp, Stroup, & Kruchko, 2012). A tumor is a mass of tissue that may be solid or filled with fluid. Tumors in the brain may cause the child to feel nauseated, vomit, or have vision prob-lems, dizziness, or trouble walking and holding things. Tumors in the spinal cord are less common for children. These types of tumors may cause motor difficul-ties and pain. These types of tumors have many possible types of presentation (see Spacca, Giordano, Donati, & Genitori, 2015). A palpable mass (tumor) is sometimes present. These tumors can be surgically removed and early detection and removal is advisable (Constantini et al., 1996). In addition to removing the tumor, preserving the functioning of the spinal cord and motor functioning is critical (Cheng et al., 2014; Spacca et al., 2015).

Prevalence

Ward et al. (2014) proposed that "…186.6 per million children and adolescents aged birth to 19 years…" are diagnosed with cancer (p. 83). Ward et al. stated that a child born in the United States has a "0.24 % chance of developing cancer before the age of 15 years…" (p. 84). The incidence of cancer is highest during infancy and drops between 5 and 9 years of age (Spector et al., 2015). Children who are Caucasian typically have higher rates of cancer compared to children in other ethnic groups (Kazak & Noll, 2015; Spector et al., 2015). Boys are more likely to be diagnosed with cancer compared to girls (Siegel et al., 2014; Spector et al., 2015). A very small percentage of childhood cancers have preventable causes.

Leukemia is the most common type of cancer faced by children (about 1/3 of cancers for children are Leukemias; Siegel et al., 2014), particularly Acute Lymphocytic Leukemias, which account for about 77 % of Leukemia cases (Siegel, Miller, & Jemal, 2015; Siegel, Naishadham, & Jemal, 2013). The next most com-mon types of cancers are cancers of the brain and nervous system (Ward et al., 2014). From 2007 to 2011 the incidence of cancer increased 0.6 % in children ages 14 and younger (Siegel et al., 2015).

Twenty-one percent of brain tumors are in one of the four lobes of the brain (frontal, parietal, occipital, or temporal lobes). Tumors of the meninges (the mem-branes covering the brain) are the most common brain tumors. Tumors in the cranial nerves (connected to the spinal cord) and spinal cord account for about 10 % of brain and spinal cord tumors. These types of tumors carry significant risk for children, in their removal and treatment (Dolecek et al., 2012).

In 2015, it was estimated that approximately 10,380 children between birth and 14 years of age will be diagnosed with cancer. Cancer is a leading cause of mortality for children (Wolfe et al., 2015). Specifically, Siegel et al. (2013) reported that cancer was the second leading cause of death, behind accidental injury, for children between the ages of 1 and 14 years who were living in the United States. In 2009, 1,320 children died of cancer (Siegel et al., 2013) and in 2015 it was estimated that 1,250 children would die from cancer (Siegel et al., 2015). Then again, more children are surviving cancer, with approximately 83 % surviving what used to be considered a terminal disease for children (Siegel et al., 2015).

Genetic and Environmental Determinants

Genetics play a role in childhood cancer, although more information is needed to explain the heritability of this illness (Miller, 2012; Spector et al., 2015). An in-depth review of the genetic determinants of cancer is beyond the scope of this chapter. Interested readers may enjoy reviewing a book entitled, *Genetics for Health Professionals in Cancer Care: From Principals to Practice*, to learn more about genetics and cancer in children (Jacobs, Robinson, & Webb, 2014).

There are several environmental risk factors for cancer. Risks for cancer include ionizing radiation and having had chemotherapy (Spector et al., 2015). Immunosuppressive drugs, such as what one might take after a transplant, have been related to cancer risk (Miller, 2012). Radiation during the early years can increase the risk for leukemia and brain cancer. Being exposed to pesticides or chemicals are risk factors (Miller, 2012; Spector et al., 2015). Other risk factors include being overweight and having genetic or immunodeficiency syndromes (Miller, 2012; Ward et al., 2014). Exposure to smoking and paint may also be risk factors for developing cancer (Ward et al., 2014). Being exposed to parental smoking has been associated with increased risk for cancer (Kazak & Noll, 2015). Advanced parental age is another risk factor (Spector et al., 2015).

Impact on Children

Children must cope with pain related to having cancer and from procedures needed to treat cancer. They also may have to endure multiple needle sticks and venipunctures. Teaching children relaxation (e.g., breathing) and imagery (thinking pleasant and happy thoughts) techniques, such as those described in Chap. 4 (*Coping with Pain*) can help them to relax when they are undergoing medical procedures. Young children may be best served by distraction (playing games, watching a funny movie, holding a favorite toy) and physical comfort as pain relief strategies, but these strategies can help older children as well. Younger children can blow bubbles to practice taking a deeper breath to relax, and the bubbles serve as distraction as well. Older children may benefit from listening to a playlist of favorite songs or playing a computer game to help distract them and help them relax, when undergoing painful procedures.

Children with cancer, who experience invasive treatments that cross the blood–brain barrier, may be especially prone to neurological and cognitive problems after cancer treatment. These children may need continued monitoring of school performance and intellectual functioning and may benefit from Individual Education Programs (IEPs) to help them do well at school. They may experience problems with attention, concentration, memory, and organizational abilities at school. They may benefit from having extra time to complete tests, special education interventions to improve attention, concentration and memory, and counseling if these problems are upsetting to the child.

Children with cancer also may feel or be isolated from their peers. They may benefit from social skills interventions to help them learn to join in play and other peer interactions and converse with others in their age group. The health educator can arrange a buddy system for a child newly diagnosed with cancer so that he or she can play with another child who has undergone a similar illness. In addition, support groups may help children find understanding friends who are coping with cancer. Children with cancer may feel awkward at school and review of ways to explain cancer to peers and let peers know that they cannot "catch" cancer may assist the child with cancer in explaining his or her condition to others. Alternately, the health educator can explain the condition to the child's peers in the classroom, and answer any medical questions, to reduce awkward moments when the child returns to school after intensive cancer treatments, such as those that involve chemotherapy and result in hair loss and other physical changes.

Late Effects: The 5-year survival rate for children who have cancer is a little over 80 %, which is very encouraging. However, there are many factors to deal with after cancer treatments. For instance, most children who survive cancer are at risk for having another type of chronic illness by the age of 40 (Robinson & Hudson, 2014). Children who are cancer survivors also may be more likely to cope with infections and they have poorer immune function due to having had cancer and often as a result of undergoing chemotherapy (Perkins et al., 2014). These problems typically emerge in young adulthood and are termed late effects.

Despite the increased survivorship about "…70 % of pediatric cancer survivors develop late effects that can be chronic or even life-threatening (e.g., infertility, cardiovascular/lung disease, renal dysfunction, severe musculoskeletal problems, endocrinopathies, second cancers, cognitive impairments." (Kazak & Noll, 2015, p. 148). The chronic medical problems known often as late effects can emerge at any time, but often occur in early adulthood. Many children with cancer do not follow recommendations for health-promoting behaviors and medical follow-up recommended by their medical team, which puts them at more risk for having more serious consequences from late effects related to cancer treatments. Children with brain tumors may be especially vulnerable to significant health risks after cancer treatments (Kazak & Noll, 2015).

Treatment of cancer usually involves using multiple chemotherapies and may involve radiation or surgical resection. This treatment creates risk for late effects (Vannatta, Salley, & Gerhardt, 2009). Although more children are surviving this disease, they are living with other chronic health problems (e.g., organ damage), pain, growth retardation, renal or reproductive problems, as well as neurological and cognitive deficits (Phillips et al., 2015; Vannatta et al., 2009). Children who have survived cancer also may experience heart problems, and cardiac toxicity is possible later in life (van der Pal et al., 2015). Another problem may be sleep disordered breathing (Ruble, George, Gallicchio, & Gamaldo, 2015). Long-term cancer survivors may experience the aforementioned late effects, which are related to decreased quality of life as well as increased mortality. Efforts need to be directed toward long-term care and planning for optimal development and quality of life for childhood cancer survivors. Long-term follow-up and assessment of child functioning is needed to understand what will support children. Medical teams need to continue to monitor physical functioning to detect problems, such as secondary malignancies and the possible emergence of many types of late effects (Vannatta et al., 2009).

Impact on Family Caregivers

Caring for a child who has cancer is complex and takes courage and caring. Caregivers, usually parents or other close family members, face many challenges. Challenges experienced by the family, especially in terms of caregiving, have increased due to shorter hospital stays and a shift in the burden of care to families. Stenberg, Ruland, and Miaskowski (2010) reviewed 192 studies focusing on caregiving for children with cancer. Their findings revealed a plethora of challenges faced by family caregivers. Some of these include challenges in caring for other children and family members, paying the bills, keeping a job, and feeling a loss of social and sometimes marital support (Stenberg et al., 2010). Other issues for family caregivers are feeling pain, fatigue, loss of sleep, decreased appetite, depression, and fear related to their child's condition. Parents who are lacking a strong social network may be at risk for feeling overwhelmed, as they do not have psychological support to express their feelings about their child nor do they have support (e.g., babysitting) to help them to care for the rest of the family. Families who are feeling extreme financial burden due to their child's chronic illness also may have parents or siblings who may be at risk for negative psychological outcomes. Accordingly, another goal for health educators working with children who have cancer is to care for the family unit, by educating caregivers about how to cope with the child's illness as well as about some of the negative psychological and behavioral outcomes they may face. Family caregivers may also benefit from support, either through support groups or internet support, to help them reduce feelings of loneliness and isolation and to provide them with outlets for speaking with other parents who are going through a similar trauma with their child.

Sulkers et al. (2015) also assessed the impact of a child's cancer on family caregivers. They examined mothers' reactions and discovered that reports of increased depression and anxiety were more commonly reported as risk factors than physical symptoms were. Reports of worry and problems with emotional functioning were higher immediately after a cancer diagnoses and decreased 3 months later. Single mothers or mothers whose only child had cancer were at greater risk for problems with emotional functioning. Sulkers et al. pointed out that having a child who was cancer-free might allow the mothers some moments away from the cancer experience, but more research is needed to examine if this is the reason for the buffering effect of having another child without cancer. Sulkers et al. stressed that education for mothers is critical and that health professionals need to assist mothers in strengthening their confidence that they can care for the medical needs of their child with cancer. In fact, because caregiver stress and emotional problems are significant, experts have recommended that health professionals consider the family, especially parents or primary caregivers, and the child with cancer as a unit of care when treating a child who has cancer (Ekstedt, Stenberg, Olsson, & Ruland, 2014).

Long et al. (2014) conducted a study examining parent perceptions of how a child's cancer affected them as parents. Parents of children with cancer were likely to endorse survey items indicating that they tended to spoil their child and worried that "bad or sad things" could happen to their child. Parents reported they wished that their child did not have to grow up so fast. Long et al. also assessed pediatric oncology professionals' views of child-rearing. Professionals reported that parents were likely to overprotect children and worry about them. Professionals indicated that parents were concerned about their children's eating habits. Pediatric professionals shared these opinions about child-rearing irrespective of child age range. On the other hand, parental responses did not indicate that they felt that they were overprotecting their child, and thus Long et al. surmised that parents may be paying attention to professionals' advice not to treat their child differently because of his or her chronic illness. Long et al. also stated that pediatric professionals may overgeneralize beliefs about parenting practices. It will be beneficial for health professionals to learn about individual family's parent–child relations and parenting practices before making conclusions that a child is overprotected. This study was cross-sectional in nature (this means that surveys were completed at only one point in time) and few children of color were recruited, and therefore further research will be necessary to see if differences in parent–professional beliefs are similar over time and for parents of children of color.

Assessment

Assessment of children with cancer should involve a complex assessment of child psychological functioning and school abilities. Referral to a pediatric or child health psychologist for assessment of intellectual functioning and educational abilities is recommended. Working with the child's teachers and schools to gain an accurate picture of the child's educational abilities over the course of his or her school career is important, as school absences and late effects may hinder the child's academic performance. Some children who have cancer may benefit from educational planning (e.g., having an IEP) or having a 504 plan to ensure they receive and have time to complete missed assignments. Continued assessment of intellectual and school achievement on an annual or bi-annual basis is important to ensure that the child is maintaining his or her academic performance as he or she copes with cancer. Interviewing the child and family to determine his or her emotional and social functioning is important, as depression, anxiety, and isolation can be recurrent problems for children who have cancer or are in remission from their disease.

Medications

Children with cancer often receive many types of treatments, such as chemotherapies, steroids, and surgical removal of cancer (tumors). A review of the complex chemotherapies and medical treatments is beyond the scope of this chapter and interested readers are referred to medical references (see Voûte, Barrett, Bloom, Lemerle, & Neidhardt, 2012 for example) and papers developed by pediatric oncologists. Pediatric oncologists are pediatricians specializing in the treatment of cancer.

Adherence to Medical Regimens

Adherence to medical recommendations is very important for children who have cancer. If they do not participate in treatment and follow their medical regimen, the impact of their disease is life-threatening (Kazak & Noll, 2015). Unfortunately, over 50 % of survivors do not attend their cancer-related medical appointments after treatment has ended. This can be devastating if children develop late effects—or negative health outcomes and problems related to having cancer and being treated for cancer (Brier, Schwartz, & Kazak, 2014). Moreover, following a healthy lifestyle—with a healthy diet, not smoking and plenty of exercise—is critical to survivors to ensure their health in the long run, and many need education and morale boosts so that they understand and can follow a very healthy lifestyle during and after their cancer treatment.

Ensuring that parents and children understand all aspects of medical recommendations is essential, and health educators can play a key role in ensuring that medical recommendations meet the health literacy level of parents. Health literacy is defined by this author as parents' abilities to understand the health implications of the doctor's instructions and understand the steps that need to be taken in order to administer the medical recommendations for their child. Arranging meetings with parents after diagnostic meetings may be helpful, as during initial diagnostic meetings parents are dealing with shock, denial and grief that may limit their abilities to listen to what the doctors are telling them. Having a follow-up meeting to go over medical recommendations can greatly improve parents' health literacy. It can also allow them a chance to express their feelings of grief regarding their child's diagnosis. The health educator can establish schedules, using calendars that are easy to follow, which may assist parents in understanding the "big picture." The health educator can work with parents to develop a plan for ensuring that they are able to keep track of medical appointments and complicated medication schedules. Ensuring that there is child care for long appointments can be helpful, as appointments with pediatric oncologists can be long (over 1 h in length). Helping the child tolerate pain and improving family and child spirits may provide the child and family with the resilience needed to engage in the chemotherapy and a complex treatment regimen (with appointments and medication schedules).

Psychological and Social Functioning of Children with Cancer

Acute Lymphblastic Leukemia (ALL) is the most common cancer during childhood, and children with ALL may be at risk for depression and anxiety and after treatment they may not show age-related progression of gains in cognitive functioning (Vannatta et al., 2009). Children who have survived brain tumors also may experience depression and anxiety. Late effects are also associated with social difficulties and children who have survived cancer may withdraw from others or experience peer victimization.

Children who have recovered from cancer may experience posttraumatic stress as they cope with remembering a life-threatening disease and painful and invasive treatment procedures (Vannatta & Gerhardt, 2003). Hence, children may have memories that are scary and intrusive, which cause them to "relive" treatments and surgeries. Children may recall painful experiences and being separated from their family members. Children may benefit from counseling to help them cope with stressful memories and related fears that their cancer could recur. Having experienced cancer may isolate children from peers and children who have survived cancer may have difficulty with their adolescent development and attachments with others, including the development of age-appropriate romantic relationships. Additionally, some children who have survived cancer may exhibit risky behaviors during adolescence, such as substance use. Others may be at risk for being "repressive" and holding back from adolescent experiences as they perceive themselves as being very vulnerable to health problems (Vannatta & Gerhardt, 2003).

According to experts from the Children's Oncology Group, children with ALL participate in long-term treatment with multiple types of chemotherapy agents and corticosteroids, which can impact their emotional and behavioral functioning (as well as cognition; Myers et al., 2014). Members of the Children's Oncology group conducted a prospective, longitudinal study of children with ALL who did not receive radiation treatments of their brains (in their cranial regions). They assessed several factors or variables including: child anxiety and depression, child behavioral functioning, and family functioning. They also examined family coping and child physical functioning. Their findings suggested that child anxiety was high the first month after diagnosis, but reverted to more "normal" levels after 6 and 12 months. Children were likely to experience feelings of depression during the first year of treatment; however, not all children's reports were scored at a clinically significant level (a level of sadness that would warrant diagnosis). Worse physical functioning (pain) was related to more reports of depression, but not anxiety. If family coping and functioning were poor, children also were more likely to report feelings of anxiety or depression (Myers et al., 2014). Those children who lacked social support were more likely to experience depression. Moreover, children who were depressed or anxious at 1 month after treatment began were more likely to remain anxious and depressed at 6 and 12 months. Thus, those working with children with cancer should assess children's anxiety and depression levels and follow their functioning over time to monitor their mental health and determine if referral is needed. It is noteworthy, however, that a majority of children who do survive cancer and their families are very resilient, and it is a subset that experiences clinically important levels of psychological distress (Brier et al., 2014).

Rodriguez et al. (2012) studied stress in children, ages 5–17 years, with cancer. Children in their sample, between the ages of 10 and 17 years, provided information about their stressors and their parents also provided similar information. The mean age of children in the sample was 10 years, 6 months (with a standard deviation of about 4 years). Children and parents completed several surveys. Answers provided by children and their parents were grouped into several areas that indicated concerns they had including: (a) uncertainty about the future and about the child's cancer, (b) changes in daily functioning (e.g., missing school), and (c) physical changes and effects due to treatment (e.g., feeling sick from treatment, worried about changes in the way I look). Parents and children also completed a survey to assess their stress. The most significant stressors for children appeared to be related to disruptions in daily functioning. Hence, not being able to do what they used to do was very stressful for children (Rodriguez et al.). Mothers, fathers, and children tended to agree about the types of stresses the children were experiencing, although mothers reported higher stress for children compared to fathers and the children themselves. For children, feelings of uncertainty about cancer and significant physical effects of having cancer were related to traumatic stress. It is worth mentioning that this study used surveys to examine perceptions, and this information can be valuable; however, observations of child functioning would also yield important data.

Treatment and Research About Interventions for Children with Cancer

Many children who have cancer enroll in clinical trials based on research protocols developed by the Children's Oncology Group (COG; Kazak & Noll, 2015). Specifically,
the,

> "COG includes over 200 institutions in the United States, Canada, Australia, and New Zealand and assures that children receive the same medical care on the same protocols across treatment centers. The majority of children (55 %–65 %) under the age of 14 participate in clinical trial research studies." (Kazak & Noll, 2015, p. 147).

Treatment typically involves administration of chemotherapy or several types of chemotherapy and treatment with corticosteroids. Children may be hospitalized to receive chemotherapy treatments. Children who receive chemotherapy may have weakened immune systems and their immune system is also weakened by their cancer; as a result, they may be vulnerable to infections. Thus, children may be hospitalized for treatment of infections, such as pneumonia. As mentioned, more children are surviving cancer, with over 80 % being survivors. Kazak and Noll (2015) stated that surviving was living 2 years after chemotherapy treatment had ended or at least 5 years since time of diagnosis.

Children also may receive stem cell transplantation and may be hospitalized when they receive a bone marrow transplant. A bone marrow transplant involves infusing healthy stem cells into the child's body to suppress the child's cancer and support new bone marrow growth (https://www.nlm.nih.gov/medlineplus/ency/article/003009.htm downloaded December 20, 2015). Bone marrow is the tissue inside your bones that produces blood cells. Stem cells are cells in the bone marrow that produce blood cells. A bone marrow transplant allows new blood cells to fight the cancer cells that have been growing "out of control."

Information on medical assessment and treatment of cancer is very complex. A detailed review is beyond the scope of this chapter. One possible referral source is the Children's Oncology Group webpage (https://www.childrensoncologygroup.org/). The Children's Oncology Group has developed a book, entitled, "The Family Handbook, Second Edition," that was funded by the St. Baldrick's Foundation (https://www.childrensoncologygroup.org/). The St. Baldrick's Foundation raises funds to assist those with cancer and is a great resource for health professionals (http://www.stbaldricks.org/filling-the-funding-gap; downloaded October 5, 2015). Another critical source for learning about medical treatment of cancer is the National Cancer Institute's Research Tested Programs website with an index of programs (http://rtips.cancer.gov/rtips/index.do). The Cancer Control Planet is another government website that has information about cancer treatment (http://cancercontrolplanet.cancer.gov/) and the National Cancer Institute has critical information tailored for children (http://ctep.cancer.gov/MajorInitiatives/Pediatric_Preclinical_Testing_Program.htm; downloaded October 5, 2015).

Ruland, Hamilton, and Schjødt-Osmo (2009) reviewed research on childhood cancer. Their study included both review papers and research papers about children's reactions to cancer. They reported that childhood cancer could be underdiagnosed and undertreated. Children reported many problems related to having cancer throughout their diagnosis, treatment process, and after treatment was over. Some of the symptoms included: fatigue, pain, feeling listless, changes in mood and behaviors, depression, anxiety, uncertainty about illness outcomes, fear, and feelings of stigma related to being the "child with cancer." Having cancer could be likened to a roller coaster experience where children and parents experienced a wealth of different emotions that recycled and heightened or lessened in intensity throughout the course of the disease. The multiple hospitalizations and procedures the children often faced, only served to heighten the dips and turns of this roller coaster experience. One possible resource for those interested in counseling children with pediatric cancer includes articles on psychosocial treatment of children with cancer in the journal entitled, *"Pediatric Blood and Cancer."* In their article in the *American Psychologist*, Kazak and Noll (2015) also outline the role of the pediatric psychologist or counselor in working with children who have cancer.

Children who have battled their disease for a longer period may experience high levels of distress and significant pain and fatigue. For example, Wolfe et al. (2015; PediQuest Study) examined the perceptions of 104 children or adolescents (patients were 2 years or older through the adolescent years) with cancer whose parents had decided not to pursue treatment, or where children had at least a 2-week history of progressive or recurrent cancer, or children had cancer that was not responsive to treatment. Multiple measurements of child reports of symptoms were assessed and patients were experiencing increased levels of pain, fatigue, drowsiness, problems sleeping, and irritability. Children receiving high-intensity cancer treatments were more likely to report negative physical symptoms, such as those named in the preceding sentence. Being female, having a brain tumor, having undergone recent cancer treatment, or having an exacerbation of the disease were risk factors for increased levels of distress and negative symptoms such as pain and fatigue. These authors also pointed out that children and families experience uncertainty about disease control and progression, which can heighten distress for some patients. Additionally, they found that more mild treatment in the final 12 weeks of a child's life was typically related to improved psychological well-being of the child. Thus, they recommended that providers be open to courses of mild treatment for patients, if it was medically indicated that this might be an acceptable course of action.

Children experiencing cognitive delays and late effects after cancer treatment may benefit from attentional retraining, techniques to improve memory, and other interventions to help them in areas where they are experiencing cognitive deficits. Butler and Mulhern (2005) reviewed literature showing that children benefitted from adaptations of interventions similar to those used with adults who have suffered brain damage. In their review, Butler and Mulhern noted that an extensive neuropsychological assessment (extensive tests of cognitive functioning) are needed to assess areas of delay and determine areas where intervention is needed to help improve cognitive deficits. After this the child participates in massed practice to improve attention, memory, and organizational skills as well as communication and academic skills. The child participates in drills to learn academic material during practice sessions and also learns memory strategies to boost memory skills. The educational environment can be modified so that the child can complete assignments on a computer, receive handouts that review lecture information (so that the child does not have to rely on his or her notes from the lecture session), and receive extended time on tests. In a national, randomized study with a control group, Butler et al. (2008) examined the impact of attention and memory training on child functioning. Children participated in intense training sessions (20, 2-h weekly sessions) to improve their attention, concentration, and memory skills (using computer games, problem-solving, drills and practice with trained educators). Results indicated that children showed improved attention, memory and academic performance after participating in this intervention. Kesler, Lacayo, and Jo (2011) conducted a pilot study where they assessed the impact of computer training for children who were showing skills deficits after receiving cancer treatment. Results of their pilot study demonstrated that children who participated in an 8 week computer training to improve their processing speed did show gains in their memory skills, cognitive flexibility, and processing speed.

Not all studies have shown that children demonstrate gains in memory and other cognitive skills after participating in computer training. For instance, Palmer et al. (2014) delivered a computer program as a prophylactic treatment for children with medulloblastoma (a brain tumor located in the cerebellum) who were actively receiving treatment for their cancer. Children participated in a reading decoding program that they could complete on their own (it was recommended that children complete 30 sessions). Many children did not complete the recommended treatment, and the authors concluded that this might have occurred because the children were very involved in difficult cancer treatments. There was not a difference in functioning for children assigned to the treatment group and those assigned to a "standard of care" control group, where children received,

> ...the current standard of care with regard to educational services from the hospital School Program. Patients who are of school age (in this type of program) attend up to three 1-h sessions per week with a licensed teacher... the goal of these sessions is to allow the patient to complete assignments using books and activities provided by the patient's community school. (p. 452)

Children in the treatment group participated in this type of programming as well as having an opportunity to complete computer training to improve their reading skills. The treatments for cancer and the many hospital visits may have precluded some children from participating in the additional computer activities. The authors felt that this type of intervention needs further exploration rather than "waiting for a child to fail" as he or she experiences late effects from cancer and its treatment.

Interventions for the child and his or her family are also found in the literature. Svavarsdottir and Sigurdardottir (2013) examined the effectiveness of a conversation intervention for families of children and adolescents participating in cancer treatment. This intervention was termed the Family Therapeutic Conversation Intervention (FAM-TCI), which was designed to give support to primary caregivers of the child. Nurses worked with caregivers asking therapeutic questions to assist them in developing interventions that would enrich family functioning and well-being. Offering praise and drawing on family strengths were key components of the intervention. Nurses also reviewed and praised parents for ways in which they were "handling the situation well." The nurses' therapeutic questions were a critical component of the intervention, intended to encourage parents' problem-solving. Parents or caregivers, who spoke with the nurses, reported higher family and emotional support after working with the nurses. The caregivers reported better family functioning and family communication about emotional issues after participating in conversations with nurses. However, the caregivers' spouses did not indicate the same strong support, indicating that there were differences in partners' perceptions of the intervention. This was a very practical intervention, and more research will be needed to determine if therapeutic conversations by nurses and other members of the medical team are perceived as supportive. Children in the sample for this study were newly diagnosed with cancer, which restricted the sample to a high-risk group, as the time immediately after diagnosis may be very stressful. Future studies examining whether therapeutic conversations have the same high benefit after the child and family have been coping with the child's cancer for months or years will need to be conducted to determine whether this type of intervention is as helpful for families that have been dealing with a child's cancer for longer periods of time.

Brier et al. (2014) reviewed studies providing health behavior and psychosocial interventions for child cancer survivors. These researchers also reviewed neurocognitive interventions, but since the effectiveness of these types of interventions was previously discussed, the focus in these paragraphs is to present information about Brier et al.'s review of interventions to impact behavioral and psychological functioning of children. These researchers used a quality assessment tool from the Effective Public Health Practice Project which allows reviewers to judge studies based on whether there was a control group (i.e., group that did not participate in treatment), whether confounding factors (other factors that could have influenced study outcomes) were assessed, whether experimenters were blind to study hypotheses (i.e., they did not know about research questions for the study), and whether the integrity of the delivery of the intervention was assessed (i.e., did the researchers assess whether the intervention was delivered according to plan or according to the manual?).

These researchers found several studies where interventions were targeted at improving health behaviors, and several of these were randomized-controlled trials (this means that participants were randomly assigned to be in either the intervention group or a control group [typically waiting for later treatment]; Brier et al., 2014). The majority of the researchers used one-on-one counseling tailored to goals for individual children. Areas of goals for the children included increased engagement in physical activity, eating healthy, and reducing health risk behaviors (e.g., smoking, drinking). Interventions were aimed at improving children's social competence, problem-solving and decision-making, well-being, stress, and emotional and behavioral problems. Again, one-on-one and group counseling was used with children. Interventions included: (a) teaching children positive self-talk, (b) how to reframe or "rethink" negative thinking patterns [into more positive thinking patterns], (c) relaxation skills, (d) teaching children to seek information about their health, as well as (e) communication and (f) problem-solving skills. Furthermore, Brier et al. found improvements in behavioral and emotional functioning of children, reduced stress, and improved social interactions and positive relationships with others. They concluded that the interventions to improve children's behavioral and psychosocial functioning were successful. It is noteworthy that most of the studies that were reviewed had adolescents and children in the same sample, and since samples were small, it is difficult to pinpoint how developmental differences (differences based on the children's age levels) could have impacted study results. Brier et al. did suggest that participants valued convenient interventions, and that interventions delivered by telephone and internet were important to explore.

As previously mentioned, children who are recovering from cancer may cope with significant stress which can involve intrusive thoughts and trauma related to having cancer and undergoing cancer treatments. Kazak et al. (2004) developed a 1-day, intensive intervention to help adolescents cope with trauma related to having cancer. This program was entitled the, "Surviving Cancer Competently Intervention Program." Although this intervention was delivered primarily with adolescents (participants were between 11 and 19 years of age), it is possible to adapt this intervention for younger children. Separate groups were provided for mothers, fathers, children with cancer, and their siblings. Family groups were also provided, and family groups allowed family members to share their feelings with others that might be going through similar events. The intervention consisted of four sessions: (a) how cancer impacts the child and family, (b) coping skills training, (c) ideas for "getting on with life," and (d) "pulling it together." The first session addressed how distressing memories about the child's cancer and its treatment impacted the child and family. The second session involved problem-solving and reframing negative thinking related to cancer experiences. Participants were taught to focus on the controllable and the positive aspects of distressing memories. The third session focused on how cancer influenced the family "today" and several inter-family groups were conducted to allow families to process feelings. The fourth session allowed families to meet and discuss what they gained from participating and how they could apply what they had experienced to their daily lives to improve family functioning. Family members learned to respond to other family member's distress and put "cancer in its place" as the family moved forward. Results of the evaluation of this program showed that children and adolescents experienced reductions in arousal in response to events that reminded them of their cancer experience. The counseling also resulted in reductions in intrusive traumatic thoughts for fathers of cancer survivors. Kazak et al. (2004) noted that mothers seemed particularly resilient and perhaps this was why results did not indicate improved functioning for mothers. Some distressed families did drop out of the intervention, and therefore making the intervention shorter and more accessible to families may improve outreach for distressed families. Or, it may be that distressed families benefit from individually oriented counseling to help them express stress and learn problem-solving and positive self-talk to help them cope with cancer-related trauma.

Helping a Child to Die. Some children with cancer die. A key role for health professionals is to support the child and family in having a meaningful life and honor their wishes throughout the treatment process, and this includes end-of-life care. The child may benefit from participating in the Make-A-Wish Program (http:// wish.org/about-us; accessed October 6, 2015) or other similar programs for children with life-threatening chronic illnesses, should his or her disease be life-threatening. The child can have a wish, such as a trip to Disneyland, which is granted by the program. This author has seen these trips work wonders in raising the child's and the family's spirits and in bolstering their resilience. Another role would be to refer the child to a hospice or palliative care team at a children's hospital. These professionals have expertise in end-of-life care and can help parents and children to process grief, review happy memories, and these teams have great experience in honoring wishes of how a child and family wants the child to die.

Working with a child who is dying is very difficult, and the health professional should have support for him- or herself, in order to process his or her own feelings of sadness and loss. The child and family members may experience many feelings related to the impending death, including anger, grief, denial, bargaining with a higher power to make the child well, shock, and acceptance (Kübler-Ross, [forward by I. Byock], 2014). The Elizabeth Kübler-Ross Foundation (http://www.ekrfoundation.org/ accessed October 6, 2015) has wonderful information for health professionals interested in learning more about helping others with grief and loss related to the death of a loved one. Referral to psychologists or mental health professionals may also be an important part of end-of-life care, and these professionals can assist family members in dealing with the stages of bereavement before and after the child's death. A goal for the health professional is to help family members make meaning of the loss, as they remember the child and continue to develop as a family as they move forward with their lives. Siblings may be at risk for grief reactions and trauma when a brother or sister has cancer, so it is important to remember to assess sibling mental health and make referrals as needed.

Role of Health Educators

Roles for health educators may vary, depending on the roles of others on the medical team working with the child as well as the psychological and behavioral functioning of the child and the family. The health educator can provide information about the illness and link the child and family to other supports, such as support groups or peer mentors. In addition, many children and their parents are coping with grief related to the loss of children being able to participate in "normal childhood" experiences. The health educator can be a supportive "sounding board" as the child and family deal with losses related to having this illness and its complex treatment. Hocking et al. (2014) highlighted the fact that the treatments are traumatic for the parents and timing the intervention so that parents can absorb intervention messages can be important to the success of the intervention.

The health educator may also serve as a liaison with the school to help the child make up missed school work. If the child misses many school days related to hospital stays, the health educator can help to design re-entry programs that help a child complete missed school work and become re-integrated into the school routine and classroom. Another possible role, especially if the child is younger, is to work to explain the child's cancer to his or her classmates, if the child is experiencing stigma or isolation in the classroom. Screening the child for depression and anxiety as well as other psychological and behavioral problems, and making referrals as needed is an important task for health educators.

In some cases, a role is helping the child and his or her family to cope with the child's impending death. This can be extremely stressful and support for the health professional as he or she fills this critical role may be important. Helping the child learn to cope with pain by teaching the child to use behavioral strategies, such as relaxation, and cognitive strategies, such as imagery, may be another critical role. Siblings of children with cancer may feel bereft and may be experiencing grief. They may also miss their parents, if their parents must be highly involved in the care of the child who has cancer. Developing support groups for siblings or engaging in supportive meetings with siblings where they can discuss their feelings and concerns may be another important role for health educators.

Case Study

Misty is a 4-year-old girl with ALL. Her father works as an independent trucker, driving across states to deliver produce and other materials to grocery store chains. Her mother is a homemaker. The family lives nearby relatives on her mother's side of the family. Misty has attended preschool and gets along well with other children in her class and with her two teachers. The family attends church on Sundays and enjoys the support of family and friends from their religious community.

Misty was diagnosed with ALL 6 months ago. She was feeling tired and her body hurt all the time. Her pediatrician took a blood draw and then began collaborating with other pediatricians at the nearby children's hospital. Over the course of their collaboration, they discovered that Misty had ALL. After meeting with the specialists at the children's hospital, Misty's parents decided on an aggressive treatment involving several types of chemotherapy and corticosteroids. Misty has been participated in treatment for 5½ months. She goes to the hospital to receive chemotherapy. She has lost patches of hair and has many bald spots. She is on a fairly heavy dose of corticosteroids and has developed a very "puffy" appearance, especially in her face, which is known as having "cushingoid" features. Due to the heavy dose of chemotherapies and corticosteroids, Misty has experienced some changes in mood, with tearful outbursts and tantrums. Recently, she has begun wetting the bed at night. She had been completely potty-trained. She has become very attached to her mother and often uses "baby-talk," babbling and cooing to her mother.

Her mother is very distraught with Misty's behavior and has often cried most of the night, according to Misty's father. Misty's mother has had difficulty sleeping, has lost weight, and is sad most of the time, most days of the week. She continually worries about the future. Misty's mother and her father are very, very protective of Misty. She is no longer playing with her friends in the neighborhood for fear that she might become hurt. She does wear a mask for some time after chemotherapy treatments as her immune system is weakened considerably after receiving treatment.

The oncology team at the children's hospital noticed Misty's mother's sadness, her parents' tendencies to overprotect her, and have heard Misty's mother mention the regression (returning to behavior when she was a younger child) in Misty's behaviors. After a recent team meeting, the oncology team decided to refer Misty and her mother to see a health educator and child psychologist who work with the oncology team. Misty's mother made an appointment with both professionals.

The health educator worked with Misty's mother to educate her about her child's symptoms and how the chemotherapy would impact her child's behavior. The health educator realized the symptoms of depression being displayed by Misty's mother and arranged a referral for her mother to participate in counseling, with an adult counselor, to assist her in coping with grief and depression related to her child's cancer. The health educator also worked to educate Misty's mother and father about the fact that after Misty's period of wearing the mask was over she could play with other children. The health educator taught Misty's parents that she needed to live a normal life and gain social support. Treating their daughter as very fragile was actually heightening Misty's anxiety and tendencies to act younger than her years. The health educator also referred Misty's parents to a support group for parents of children with cancer.

Misty's mother also made an appointment for the family to speak with the child health psychologist or pediatric psychologist who worked with the oncology team. The pediatric psychologist asked to meet with Misty's parents first, so that she could better understand what was happening. The session with the pediatric psychologist began with her taking a careful history of Misty's birth and psychological and behavioral functioning. Similar to the health educator, the pediatric psychologist noted that Misty needed to play and gain developmentally appropriate experiences when she was well enough to interact with others and it was medically "cleared" for her to play with other children. The pediatric psychologist mentioned to Misty's parents that over 80 % of children with ALL are cured or have long periods of remission. The psychologist then stated that children need to learn social skills so that they can be ready to enter kindergarten. The pediatric psychologist explained that Misty's parents were being overprotective and treating her as a vulnerable child. And, although this was very understandable, it was limiting chances for Misty to gain social and play experiences that would spur her development. Misty's parents gravitated toward the notion of a vulnerable child, and had a chance to discuss their fears and grief over her diagnosis with the pediatric psychologist.

Misty's mother also mentioned that she was benefitting from her own counseling sessions and was now sleeping better and was eating regular meals (although she still was not eating much). Misty's mother was learning ways to express her feelings and cope with her feelings of grief and her shock at the intensive nature of the medical treatments for Misty in her sessions with her counselor.

After discussing Misty's mother's trauma, the pediatric psychologist moved to discuss the fact that Misty might also be experiencing trauma related to her medical treatments. The pediatric psychologist explained that Misty, like many children who have experienced trauma, was returning to earlier (an earlier developmental stage) behaviors with the baby-talk and bed-wetting. The pediatric psychologist was able to work with Misty's mother and father to talk about their extreme worries about their child's regression in behavior. The psychologist encouraged them to ignore baby-talk and praise Misty when she "talked like a big girl." After checking with the medical team to make sure that Misty was physically normal, in terms of bladder function, the psychologist worked with Misty's parents to develop a "dry all night" reward chart with prizes for those nights she did not wet her bed. These interventions did meet with success and Misty thrived on attention and rewards for her positive behaviors.

The pediatric psychologist was pleased to learn that Misty was coping well with venipunctures for chemotherapy and other needle sticks. Misty had a great relationship with the oncology team, which was another strength, which further bolstered her parents' confidence and feelings of security over the hospital being the "right place" for Misty's cancer treatments. Misty's parents' relationship was stronger and they were communicating regularly to support each other, which the pediatric psychologist believed was another strong sign in favor of good family coping.

The pediatric psychologist scheduled a follow-up meeting with Misty's parents to determine their progress on not treating her as being so very vulnerable and helping her have opportunities to socialize with others. They also planned to discuss Misty's parents' perceptions of the support group that they were going to attend in the near future. The church community and religion continued to be a support for Misty's parents and prayer was significantly bolstering her mother's and father's coping. The pediatric psychologist aimed to establish a strong and supportive relationship with Misty's parents so that she could be there for them when needed and assist them in processing feelings of grief and trauma related to Misty's cancer diagnosis and treatments. Furthermore, the pediatric psychologist planned to meet with Misty for play therapy sessions to support Misty as she copes with the various stages of her illness. Through the play sessions the pediatric psychologist would conduct an ongoing developmental assessment to determine Misty's progress in dealing with disease-related trauma and her adjustment to her chronic illness.

Summary

This chapter reviewed information about childhood cancer and managing psychological issues for children who are undergoing treatment or who have survived cancer. Children with cancer can experience serious health problems when they are older and thus must take care of themselves after receiving treatment. They need to eat healthy and reduce risk behaviors. In addition, psychologically, children can experience feelings of depression and isolation, and therefore some may benefit from receiving treatment for these issues. Children may experience late effects, which often involve problems with attention, concentration, and memory and children may benefit from receiving treatments similar to those offered to others with brain injuries (e.g., computer-based training) that assists children in building memory, attention, concentration, and organizational skills.

Health educators can help educate the child and his or her family about medical changes and psychosocial outcomes for children who have experienced cancer. Health educators can promote positive development in children and families and support those families and children who are functioning well, as many are very resilient. Additionally, health educators can assist with school re-entry programming and helping the child become involved in social activities with peers. Teaching parents and children to think positively about cancer memories and allowing them to express and cope with the stressors they have experienced are roles for health educators. If the child is experiencing significant depression or trauma related to cancer recovery, referral to a licensed counselor may be indicated. Individual and family interventions, which involve counseling and support, that are inexpensive and easy to administer, perhaps though telephone sessions, may be experienced positively by families and be a mechanism to reach families who might have difficulty attending hospital- or clinic-based counseling sessions.

Exercises/Review Questions

1. What are late effects for children who survive cancer and its treatment?
2. What are some psychological consequences that might be faced by childhood cancer survivors who are not adjusting well after cancer treatment?
3. In your view, what would be an ideal family-level intervention for parents of children who have survived cancer? What would help parents deal with their feelings of trauma and stress related to watching their child go through chemotherapy, in your opinion?
4. Many families have difficulty adhering to medical regimens and with keeping appointments (i.e., follow-up visits or "well checks" after their child has received intensive interventions). What would be some strategies for encouraging parents to (1) follow medical regimens and (2) keep appointments after intensive interventions have been completed?
5. Let's imagine a case. The child (an 8-year-old girl) has completed chemotherapy and is feeling very self-conscious about returning to her classroom. How would you explain her treatment to peers in the classroom and help her re-integrate or re-enter school?

Key Concepts

Acute Lymphoblastic Leukemia
Late effects
Intrusive traumatic memories
Make-A-Wish Program
Elizabeth Kubler Ross
Stages of loss/grief
Impact on caregivers
Children's Oncology Group
Common treatments for cancer
Reframing negative thinking
Surviving Cancer Competently Intervention Program

References

Brier, M. J., Schwartz, L. A., & Kazak, A. E. (2014). Psychosocial, health-promotion, and neuro-cognitive interventions for survivors of childhood cancer: A systematic review. *Health Psychology, 34*(2), 130–148. doi:10.1037/hea0000119.

Butler, R. W., Copeland, D. R., Fairclough, D. L., Mulhern, R. K., Katz, E. R., Kazak, A. E., … Sahler, O. J. Z. (2008). A multicenter, randomized clinical trial of a cognitive remediation program for childhood survivors of a pediatric malignancy. *Journal of Consulting and Clinical Psychology, 76*(3), 367–378. doi:10.1037/0022-006X.76.3.367.

Butler, R. W., & Mulhern, R. K. (2005). Neurocognitive interventions for children and adolescents surviving cancer. *Journal of Pediatric Psychology, 30*(1), 65–78. doi:10.1093/jpepsy/jsi017.

Cheng, J. S., Ivan, M. E., Stapleton, C. J., Quinones-HinoJosa, A., Gupta, N., & Auguste, K. I. (2014). Intraoperative changes in transcranial motor evoked potentials and somatosensory evoked potentials predicting outcome in children with intramedullary spinal cord tumors. *Journal of Neurosurgery Pediatrics, 13*(6), 591–599. doi:10.3171/2014.2.PEDS1392.

Constantini, S., Houten, J., Miller, D. C., Freed, D., Ozek, M. M., Rorke, L. B., … Epstein, F. J. (1996). Intramedullary spinal cord tumors in children under the age of 3 years. *Journal of Neurosurgery, 85*(6), 1036–1043.

Dolecek, T. A., Propp, J. M., Stroup, N. E., & Kruchko, C. (2012). CBTRUS statistical report: Primary brain and central nervous system tumors diagnosed in the United States in 2005–2009. *Neuro-Oncology, 14*(Supplement 5), v1–v49. doi:10.1093/neuonc/nos218.

Ekstedt, M., Stenberg, U., Olsson, M., & Ruland, C. M. (2014). Health care professionals' perspectives of the experiences of family caregivers during in-patient cancer care. *Journal of Family Nursing, 20*(4), 462–486. doi:10.177/1074840714556179.

Hocking, M. C., Kazak, A. E., Schneider, S., Barkman, D., Barakat, L. P., & Deatrick, J. A. (2014). Parent perspectives on family-based psychosocial interventions in pediatric cancer: A mixed-methods approach. *Supportive Care in Cancer, 22*(5), 1287–1294. doi:10.1007/s00520-013-2083-1.

Jacobs, C., Robinson, L., & Webb, P. (Eds.). (2014). *Genetics for health professionals in cancer care: From principles to practice*. Oxford, England: Oxford University Press.

Kazak, A. E., Alderfer, M. A., Streisand, R., Simms, S., Rourke, M. T., Barakat, L. P., … Cnaan, A. (2004). Treatment of posttraumatic stress symptoms in adolescent survivors of childhood cancer and their families: A randomized clinical trial. *Journal of Family Psychology, 18*(3), 493–504. doi:10.1037/0893-3200.18.3.493.

Kazak, A. E., & Noll, R. B. (2015). The integration of psychology in pediatric oncology research and practice: Collaboration to improve care and outcomes for children and families. *American Psychologist, 70*(2), 146–158. doi:10.1037/a0035695.

Kesler, S. R., Lacayo, N. J., & Jo, B. (2011). A pilot study of an online cognitive rehabilitation program for executive function skills in children with cancer-related brain injury. *Brain Injury, 25*, 101–112. doi:10.1016/j.clbc.2013.02.004.

Kübler-Ross, E. with a forward by I. Byock. (2014). *On death and dying: What the dying have to teach doctors, nurses, clergy, and their own families.* New York, NY: Scribner. (Original book published in 1969).

Long, K. A., Keeley, L., Reiter-Purtill, J., Vannatta, K., Gerhardt, C. A., & Noll, R. B. (2014). Child-rearing in the context of childhood cancer: Perspectives of parents and professionals. *Pediatric Blood & Cancer, 61*, 326–332. doi:10.1002/pbc.24556.

Miller, R. W. (2012). Aetiology and epidemiology. In P. A. Voûte, A. Barrett, H. J. G. Bloom, J. Lemerle, & M. K. Neidhardt (Eds.), *Cancer in children: Clinical management* (pp. 3–8). New York, NY: Springer.

Myers, R. M., Balsamo, L., Lu, X., Devidas, M., Hunger, S. P., Carroll, W. L., … Kadan-Lottick, N. S. (2014). A prospective study of anxiety, depression, and behavioral changes in the first year after a diagnosis of childhood Acute Lymphoblastic Leukemia. *Cancer, 120*, 1417–1425. doi:10.1002/cncr.28578.

Palmer, S. L., Leigh, L., Ellison, S. C., Onar-Thomas, A., Wu, S., Qaddoumi, I., … Gajjar, A. (2014). Feasibility and efficacy of a computer-based intervention aimed at preventing reading decoding deficits among children undergoing active treatment for medulloblastoma: Results of a randomized trial. *Journal of Pediatric Psychology, 39*(4), 450–458. doi:10.1093/jpepsy/jsto95.

Perkins, J. L., Chen, Y., Harris, A., Diller, L., Stovall, M., Armstrong, G. T., … Sklar, C. A; On Behalf of the Childhood Cancer Society. (2014). Infections among long-term survivors of childhood and adolescent cancer: A report from the Childhood Cancer Survivor Study. *Cancer, 120*(16), 2514–2521. doi:10.1002/cncr.28763.

Phillips, S. M., Padgett, L. S., Leisenring, W. M., Stratton, K. K., Bishop, K., Krull, K. R., … Mariotto, A. B. (2015). Survivors of childhood cancer in the United States: Prevalence and burden of morbidity. *Cancer Epidemiology Biomarkers & Prevention, 24*(4), 653–663.

Robinson, L. L., & Hudson, M. M. (2014). Survivors of childhood and adolescent cancer: Life-long risks and responsibilities. *Nature Reviews Cancer, 14*(1), 61–70. doi:10.1038/nrc3634.

Rodriguez, E. M., Dunn, M. J., Zuckerman, T., Vannatta, K., Gerhardt, C. A., & Compas, B. E. (2012). Cancer-related sources of stress for children with cancer and their parents. *Journal of Pediatric Psychology, 37*(2), 185–197. doi:10.1093/jpepsy/jsro54.

Ruble, K., George, A., Gallicchio, L., & Gamaldo, C. (2015). Sleep disordered breathing risk in childhood cancer survivors: An exploratory study. *Pediatric Blood & Cancer, 62*(4), 693–697.

Ruland, C. M., Hamilton, G. A., & Schjødt-Osmo, B. (2009). The complexity of symptoms and problems experienced in children with cancer: A review of the literature. *Journal of Pain and Symptom Management, 37*(3), 403–418.

Siegel, D. A., King, J., Tai, E., Buchanan, N., Ajani, U. A., & Li, J. (2014). Cancer incidence rates and trends among children and adolescents in the United States, 2001–2009. *Pediatrics, 134*(4), 1–11. doi:10.1542/peds.2013-3926.

Siegel, R. L., Miller, K. D., & Jemal, A. (2015). Cancer statistics, 2015. *CA: A Cancer Journal for Clinicians, 65*(1), 5–29. doi:10.3322/caac.21254.

Siegel, R., Naishadham, D., & Jemal, A. (2013). Cancer statistics, 2013. *CA: A Cancer Journal for Clinicians, 63*(1), 11–30. doi:10.3322/caac.21166.

Spacca, B., Giordano, F., Donati, P., & Genitori, L. (2015). Spinal tumors in children: Long term retrospective evaluation of a series of 134 cases treated in a single unit of pediatric neurosurgery. *The Spine Journal, 15*(9), e1949–e1955. doi:10.1016/j.spinee.2015.04.012.

Spector, L. G., Pankratz, N., & Marcotte, E. L. (2015). Genetic and nongenetic risk factors for childhood cancer. *Pediatric Clinics of North America, 62*(1), 11–25.

Stenberg, U., Ruland, C. M., & Miaskowski, C. (2010). Review of the literature on the effects of caring for a patient with cancer. *Psycho-Oncology, 19*(10), 1013–1025.

Sulkers, E., Tissing, W. J., Brinksma, A., Roodbol, P. F., Kamps, W. A., Stewart, R. E., … Fleer, J. (2015). Providing care to a child with cancer: A longitudinal study on the course, predictors, and impact of caregiving stress during the first year after diagnosis. *Psycho-Oncology, 24*(3), 318–324. doi:10.1002/pon.3652.

Svavarsdottir, E. K., & Sigurdardottir, A. O. (2013). Benefits of a brief therapeutic conversation intervention for families of children and adolescents in active cancer treatment. *Oncology Nursing Forum, 40*(5), E346–E357.

van der Pal, H. J., van Dijk, I. W., Geskus, R. B., Kok, W. E., Koolen, M., Sieswerda, E., … van Dalen, E. C. (2015). Valvular abnormalities detected by echocardiography in 5-year survivors of childhood cancer: A long-term follow-up study. *International Journal of Radiation Oncology, Biology, Physics, 91*(1), 213–222.

Vannatta, K., & Gerhardt, C. A. (2003). Pediatric oncology: Psychosocial outcomes for children and families. In M. C. Roberts (Ed.), *Handbook of pediatric psychology* (3rd ed., pp. 342–357). New York, NY: Guilford.

Vannatta, K., Salley, C. G., & Gerhardt, C. A. (2009). Pediatric oncology: Progress and future challenges. In M. C. Roberts & R. G. Steele (Eds.), *Handbook of pediatric psychology* (4th ed., pp. 319–333). New York, NY: Guilford.

Voûte, P. A., Barrett, A., Bloom, H. J. G., Lemerle, J., & Neidhardt, M. K. (Eds.). (2012). *Cancer in children: Clinical management*. New York, NY: Springer.

Ward, E., DeSantis, C., Robbins, A., Kohler, B., & Jemal, A. (2014). Childhood and adolescent cancer statistics, 2014. *CA: A Cancer Journal for Clinicians, 64*(2), 83–103. doi:10.3322/caac.21219.

Wolfe, J., Orellana, L., Ullrich, C., Cook, E. F., Kang, T. I., Rosenberg, A., … Dussel, V. (2015). Symptoms and distress in children with advanced cancer: Prospective patient-reported outcomes from the PediQUEST study. *Journal of Clinical Oncology, 33*(17), 1928–1935. doi:10.1200/JCO.2014.59.1222.

Chapter 6
Autism Spectrum Disorder

Diagnosis

Two criteria are critical to the diagnosis of Autism Spectrum Disorder (ASD). These two criteria are: (1) persistent deficits in social communication and interaction and (2) restricted, repetitive interests, activities, and/or behaviors (American Psychiatric Association, 2013). Deficits in social communication and social interaction need to occur in multiple settings (such as home and school) and have a significant impact on child functioning. The restricted, repetitive patterns of behavior or interests also need to occur in multiple settings and significantly impair functioning. Examples of repetitive behaviors include hand-flapping, rocking, and spinning objects. Children with autism may experience comorbid or co-occurring problems. Chief among these co-occurring problems may be intellectual disorders, hyperactivity, anxiety, and "acting out" or aggressive behaviors (Gotham et al., 2013). Children with ASD also have significant difficulties with language. This can be termed having a "structural language disorder." A structural language disorder is defined as, "…inability to develop or understand sentences with proper grammar" (p. 58, American Psychiatric Association, 2013). When a mental health or medical professional is providing a diagnosis of ASD, he or she also needs to specify whether the child has an intellectual impairment and the level of severity of impaired functioning for the child.

Specifying Intellectual Impairment. As mentioned, the mental health provider should specify whether the ASD occurs with or without intellectual impairment. An intellectual disability is defined as significant deficits in intellectual or cognitive functioning, such as significant deficits in reasoning or abstract thinking. The intellectual deficits are accompanied by deficits in adaptive functioning. Deficits in adaptive functioning are those deficits that prevent a child from performing age appropriate tasks of daily living, such as feeding oneself, using crosswalks appropriately, communicating with others, and functioning independently at school. A

© Springer International Publishing Switzerland 2016
L. Nabors, *Medical and Mental Health During Childhood*, Springer
Series on Child and Family Studies, DOI 10.1007/978-3-319-31117-3_6

child with deficits in adaptive functioning would not be able to function at an age appropriate level (e.g., dressing and crossing the street), in order to be able to complete tasks of daily living in multiple settings, such as at school or at home.

Intellectual deficits are categorized into four levels in the DSM-5. The highest level of intellectual deficits occurs when a child is at the level of mild intellectual deficits. This is followed by moderate, severe, and profound intellectual deficits. Children with moderate deficits typically need special services at school and may not be able to complete daily living skills without some assistance. Children with mild deficits in intellectual functioning may also need assistance and support at school to complete their work and interact with peers. Children experiencing severe and profound deficits may not be able to be fully integrated into the regular classroom setting without an aide or one-on-one assistance. They are severely delayed in their academic skills and abilities to perform tasks of daily living (American Psychiatric Association, 2013).

Specifying Severity Level. There are three severity levels for specifying the support that the child with ASD needs. The first level, "level one," is classified as, "support needed," and typically children need support to attain educational milestones and develop their abilities to engage in social conversations. At "level two," which is classified as needing "substantial support," the child needs a greater level of support to function within daily environments, such as when he or she is at school and in the community. The third level, entitled, "substantial support," indicates that the child is experiencing significant impairments and needs substantial care from others to be able to function. When a child is classified as needing substantial support, the child may need care from other professionals to engage in normal life activities in addition to substantial support from parents in the home setting. These deficits will be life-long and the child will need long-term care if parents are no longer able to care for the child in the home.

It is very important to note that some have called the DSM-5 diagnosis of ASD into question (Kulage, Smaldone, & Cohn, 2014). The reason for this is because the DSM-5 diagnosis combines several previous diagnoses for children with a variety of symptoms across an array of functional levels. Some experts are concerned that the ASD diagnosis lacks the specificity it needs. Mental health professionals rely on specific diagnoses as "benchmarks" for treatment in order to refer children to programs and design intervention plans that will adequately meet children's needs. The general nature of the ASD diagnosis may make it less easy to plan and refer children with autism to the "right" level of treatment. When mental health professionals are using this diagnosis, they may need to provide a very clear description of the child's needs for treatment and intervention in the school setting. Detailed information of the child's strengths and weaknesses should be provided in order to develop appropriate intervention plans. These plans should address the child's needs in terms of remediating deficits in functioning, including the child in regular education settings with appropriate supports, and capitalizing on the child's strengths so that he or she can function more adaptively and learn new skills.

Prevalence

Approximately 1 % of the children in the United States and other countries have ASD (American Psychiatric Association, 2013). Volkmar et al. (2014) reviewed existing studies and found that "…prevalence estimated for autistic disorder range from 0.7 in 10,000 to 72.6 in 10,000…" depending on the study (p. 239). They mentioned that children with ASD exhibit a very broad array of symptoms, which may influence prevalence rates across studies. Additionally, the definition of this disorder has varied over time, and this may have influenced prevalence rates. Rates of autism have increased, and this may have occurred because the diagnosis is broader in scope or because mental health professionals are better at identifying this disorder (Kulage et al., 2014). However, another reason could account for this and consequently further research is needed to understand why the prevalence of autism is increasing.

There are sex and ethnic group differences. Rates of ASD are four times greater in boys than in girls (American Psychiatric Association, 2013; Kogan et al., 2009). Nonhispanic black children and multiracial children have lower rates of ASD than nonhispanic white children (Becerra et al., 2014; Kogan et al., 2009). However, ASD does occur in children of color. In a fairly recent study, Becerra et al. (2014) discovered that children of color with foreign-born mothers of color were at higher risk for severe levels of impairment associated with ASD compared to white children born of mothers who were natives of the United States.

Genetic and Environmental Influences

Multiple genes interact to influence the symptoms of ASD (Volkmar et al., 2014). Higher rates of autism are found in siblings and even higher concordance rates for autism are found in identical twins. Parent-level risk factors for ASD include parent age (with older maternal and paternal ages being risk factors), premature birth, and close spacing between pregnancies. Family members of children with ASD also can display problems with social communication and language development (Volkmar et al.). Other risk factors for ASD include having "older" parents, low birth weight, and fetal exposure to Valproate (American Psychiatric Association, 2013).

Impact for Children

The diagnosis of ASD is typically made when a child is either around age 2 or during the preschool years. If substantial impairment is involved, then the diagnosis may be made at younger ages (e.g., around 12–24 months of age or younger; American Psychiatric Association, 2013). Volkmar et al. (2014) discussed several features that may signal ASD in children including lack of language, inconsistent social communication or deficits in social communication, repetitive behaviors, restricted interests, and a need for sameness or resistance to change. At school age, children's repetitive behaviors may increase, which can be concerning for parents. Social and communication skills also can improve at school age, but usually lag behind those of children who are developing typically (developing normally without any medical or mental health problems).

The next paragraphs in this section describe repetitive behaviors, tendencies to repeat what others say, and information about the need for sameness and narrow interests for children with ASD. These are key features of ASD and these symptoms may impact children's abilities to communicate with others and be integrated with peers. These features also may negatively impact children's school performance. Children with ASD are likely to experience intellectual deficits and research discussing this is presented at the end of this impact section.

Stereotypies. A stereotypy (stereotypies) involves repetitive behavior, rigidly repeated in the same way, over and over (Cunningham & Schreibman, 2008). The stereotypy is not functional in nature for the individual. That is, the repetitive behavior is not socially appropriate or age appropriate. Stereotypies can involve repetitive use of language or repetitive behaviors, such as rocking, hand-flapping, or spinning objects. The fixation can involve parts of objects, such as spinning wheels on toy cars, or can even involve repeated visual stimulation, such as visual stimulation gained from turning lights on and off (watching light appear and then disappear). Stereotypic behaviors may be displayed when children have other types of disorders, such as intellectual deficits. Stereotypies can make a child "stand out," because this behavior is different from behaviors typically displayed by peers. Moreover, stereotypic behavior can interfere with the child's ability to learn. Furthermore, there is some evidence that the stereotypy may provide sensory stimulation; therefore, reinforcing it being repeated by the child (Cunningham & Schreibman). This is a fairly simplistic definition of stereotypies, as there are many possible repetitive behaviors. However, this information is presented to provide the reader with a "glimpse" of this type of behavior, which is common for many youth who have ASD.

Echolalia. Echolalia or repeating back parts of sentences ("echoing" speech) without necessarily intending to use the words for social communication is a hallmark behavior for some children with autism (Grossi, Marcone, Cinquegrana, & Gallucci, 2013). Echolalia occurs when children with ASD repeat language used by others; this repetition of language is not appropriate to the social setting or content of the conversation in the social interaction. When engaging in echolalia, the individual is not necessarily using the language for communicative value, but rather is repeating phrases he or she has heard. This can be the end of a sentence, a few words in a sentence, or one word. For example, another person could ask a child, "Do you want to have juice, milk, or water with your snack today?" Then, an individual with ASD who was engaging in echolalia might say, "Snack today. Snack today. Snack today." Another example might be if a teacher said, "Class, please take out your notebooks as we are going to write in our journal today." A child would be engaging in "echolalia" if he or she said, "Notebook. Notebook. Notebook."

Insistence on Sameness or Routine. Children with ASD may have an insistence on sameness—keeping with their routine—and have difficulty accepting change in their daily routines or the manner in which they accomplish daily tasks (Gotham et al., 2013). They may always do things in the same way; thus, it appears as if a series of rituals govern how they accomplish tasks. Children with ASD may become very upset if things are not the same. For instance, if there is a substitute teacher in the classroom and activities that the class completes are "out of order," for example, if reading time comes before math time, as child with an ASD could become very upset. Another example might be a change in a ritual, such as a method of getting dressed. For instance, if shoe strings were tied in a single rather than a double knot or if a child was asked to wear shorts instead of pants, then the child may become very upset. The child may need to eat only certain foods, eat only orange foods, and become upset if another food was introduced on his or her plate. The insistence on sameness may be related to the rigidity and tendency to repeat behaviors for children with autism. Recent research has shown that an insistence on sameness is not necessarily associated with anxiety, although when routines are broken a child with autism can appear anxious (Gotham et al.). On the other hand, a focus on sameness may serve to limit sensory input, so that when the sameness is interrupted anxiety is evident (Lidstone et al., 2014). It may be that anxiety is related to the disruption of some routines, but not others. More research will be needed to uncover the relationship between insistence on sameness, need for routine and repetitive behaviors, and anxiety and becoming upset when routines are disrupted.

Narrow Interests Limit Social Connection. Children with ASD may have very narrow interests in that they are only interested in a few things and have a lot of difficulty connecting with others outside this very narrow range of interests. For example, a child may only talk about or show interest in two or three topics. A child at a local elementary school may like to discuss maps and draw figures from a favorite cartoon, and outside of these interests may show little interest in other topics. This makes it hard to connect to other children who like to discuss a range of television shows and favorite activities. Children with ASD may have difficulty turn-taking when conversing or talking about topics that differ from their narrow range of interests making it difficult for them to connect with peers.

Intellectual Delays. Volkmar et al. (2014) proposed that approximately 85 % of persons with ASD experience intellectual disability; therefore, specification of the level of intellectual functioning is an important piece of information when providing this diagnosis. Specifically, 50 % may have severe or profound intellectual disability (which is often related to them needing continual support from others). Thirty-five percent experience mild levels of intellectual disability, whereas 20 % of individuals with autism have cognitive functioning in the normal range. For most children with ASD, their nonverbal, visually oriented, problem-solving skills are a relative strength and their verbal abilities are a relative weakness. This trend can be reversed in children with ASD who are high functioning.

Assessment of Autism Spectrum Disorders

There are many assessment tools for assessing symptoms related to ASD. In this section, one diagnostic interview and two other tools will be reviewed. The Diagnostic Interview for Social and Communication Disorders (DISCO) is a set of 14 items designed to identify critical features of autism based on the DSM-5 diagnostic criteria (Carrington et al., 2015). Eleven of the items focus on social and communication deficits that are common for youth with ASD. The other three items allow for assessment of repetitive behaviors, insistence on sameness in routines, and repetitive, ritualized patterns of verbal and nonverbal behaviors (stereotypies). Some of the items in this tool include: one-sided social approaches, not seeking comfort and not giving comfort to others, lacking emotionality, not sharing interests with others, lack of interactions with peers, echolalia, limited pattern of activities, and lack of friendships with peers (see Carrington et al., 2014 for more information about this tool). The items on this interview can be used with other information, which is gathered from interviewing parents and others such as teachers, to help identify symptoms of ASD. This tool can be used across a variety of age ranges and is especially helpful in identifying key social and communication deficits (Carrington et al., 2015).

Standardized screening of young children with ASD may reduce tendencies to overlook ASD symptoms in very young children. Herlihy et al. (2014) found that toddlers and young preschoolers who were screened using the Modified Checklist for Autism in Toddlers (M-CHAT; Robins, Fein, & Barton, 1999) and who participated in a follow-up interview and evaluation (with surveys designed to assess symptoms of ASD) were more likely to be diagnosed with developmental delays. This may allow children to receive early intervention, which can significantly improve behavioral and social functioning. The M-CHAT is a questionnaire with 23 items for parents to answer. The questions review key symptoms related to having developmental delays (being behind in terms of developmental skills) and symptoms of autism in very young children. Parents answer "yes" or "no" for each question. Children who are positive on three of the 23 items or two of six critical items are considered to be at higher risk for ASD.

The M-CHAT has been revised and is now the M-CHAT-R/F, which stands for the Modified Checklist for Autism in Toddlers with Follow-Up (Robins, Fein, & Barton, 2009; material about this screening tool is available at www.m-chat.org accessed on December 23, 2015). This measure is screening tool health professionals can use to interview parents, in order to determine if children display some symptoms consistent with ASD (Robins et al., 2014). This measure is available at www.mchatscreen.com. Parents or caregivers respond to a series of "yes" or "no" questions such as, "Does your child look you in the eye when you are talking to him or her, playing with him or her, or dressing him or her?" Other questions are, "Does your child try to copy what you do?" (for example: clap or make a funny noise when you do) and "Does your child make unusual finger movements near his or her eyes?" This measure takes less than 5 min to administer. If the child's total score is "0–2" then the child is considered to be at low risk. If the score is between "3 and 7" then risk is considered "medium." If the total score is between "8 and 20" then referral should occur. If the children screen positive, or at a level considered to be at medium or high risk for possibly having the disorder, then follow-up involves the health professional asking additional information about positive responses to questions on this screening tool. The M-CHAT-R/F is a broad measure and it should only be used for screening. A child with a positive screen would need to be referred for a comprehensive assessment before any type of diagnosis could be made. If a child is younger than 2 years of age, re-screening with the M-CHAT-R/F can occur again at 24 months of age.

The Childhood Autism Rating Scale (CARS) is a screening tool to use with children older than 2 years of age. This screening tool is now in its second version, the CARS, Second Edition, and it is available to be purchased from MHS Psychological Assessment and Services at http://www.mhs.com/product.aspx?gr=edu&prod=cars&id=overview (accessed December 23, 2015). Another outlet for accessing the CARS is http://www.wpspublish.com/store/p/2696/childhood-autism-rating-scale-second-edition-cars-2 (accessed December 23, 2015). The CARS was developed by Eric Schopler (e.g., Schopler, Reichler, DeVellis, & Daly, 1980). This measure takes about 5–10 min to administer and should be administered by a trained health professional. The "rater" for the CARS, Second Edition is the clinician or health provider and ratings for items (representing different behaviors and symptoms related to ASD) on this survey or scale are made based on the frequency, duration and "peculiarity" of the behavior or symptom (Schopler, Van Bourgondien, Wellman, & Love, 2010). The clinician rates the child's abilities to relate to people, repetitive behaviors, adaptation to change, verbal and nonverbal communication skills, emotional and intellectual functioning, and other behaviors that are typically observed in children with ASD. There are 15 items on this measure. Ratings are made on a 4-point scale (with 1 being normal and a rating of 4 being severely abnormal). There are also forms for the CARS to assess caregiver perceptions of the child's symptoms (http://www.wpspublish.com/store/p/2696/childhood-autism-rating-scale-second-edition-cars-2 accessed December 23, 2015).

Disease Management

Behavioral interventions, relying on reinforcement of communicative and adaptive behaviors and educational interventions, have a strong evidence base for improving children's functioning (Volkmar et al., 2014). Children with ASD benefit from reinforcement of appropriate behaviors. Behavioral plans to improve communication skills and reduce repetitive behaviors should be implemented, with an emphasis on replacing negative behaviors with more acceptable ones and ignoring negative behaviors or withdrawing reinforcement of negative behaviors until they diminish in frequency. Educational instruction is important to provide learning through repetition, visual tools (e.g., picture cards with symbols to spur communication or to show the child his/her daily schedule), and other special instructional interventions to improve the child's achievement at school and the child's adaptive functioning. Adaptive functioning involves skills needed to complete tasks of daily living, such as washing, dressing, and clearing plates from the table. Other adaptive skills or survival abilities include crossing the street, using a public restroom, and being able to read crosswalk signs. Children with ASD benefit from having special programming or Individualized Education Programs in place at school so that their special education needs can be addressed by experts (i.e., the special education team).

Training in communication skills, including the social use of language or sign language to improve social communication are an important components of intervention programs (Volkmar et al., 2014). Teaching the child through modeling with visual examples where needed, using reinforcers or rewards that are important to the child him- or herself, teaching in a step-by-step fashion, and using repetition and routine can be techniques that facilitate learning. As mentioned, visual schedules and verbal rehearsal of appropriate social interactions can be valuable teaching tools. Visual schedules may include steps in an activity or activities that the child will engage in throughout the day. Activities may be depicted using drawings or pictures on a card. Children with ASD often have more developed visual and spatial skills, and seeing what they are doing for the day may make it easier to transition between activities. Social scripts can also be useful. Social scripts spell out, step-by-step, the steps in a social interaction so that the child can memorize a set of social behaviors to use when interacting with others. When scripts are used the child may learn some verbal routines that teach him or her how to initiate conversation, take turns when talking to others, ask others about their interests, and engage others in conversations about topics of interest.

Parents often need to participate in training so they can learn important principles of reinforcement, shaping (rewarding step-by-step progress toward learning a behavior), and use of ignoring and redirection to alternative, age-appropriate activities. The aforementioned concepts are key principles in behavior modification and the health professional that is educating parents is advised to be well versed in this area. Parents probably will also need to reinforce the behavioral goals and skills that the child is learning at school or in other intervention settings. The parent needs to help the child practice the skills at home and in other community settings, in order for generalization of the performance of the new skills in different settings. Specifically, generalization occurs when the same new behavior or skills can be performed in different settings under different circumstances. Generalization of skills learned at school may not necessarily occur at home, unless there is practice in executing the steps of the behaviors at home. Another part of treatment may be parent support systems, through groups and buddy systems, as caregiver burden is high for parents of children with ASD.

Children with ASD may participate in "ABA training" or Applied Behavior Analysis Training. There are many web-based sources to help professionals learn about ABA and there are many training institutes (one possible "online" source http://www.appliedbehavioralstrategies.com/what-is-aba.html; accessed December

22, 2015). ABA training is typically provided by or supervised by a professional who is certified or licensed as an ABA specialist. This person is trained specifically in the use of reinforcement (use of rewards to change behavior), shaping behaviors (step-by-step learning of a behavior until it is mastered), understanding the functions of a child's behavior (i.e., factors that start and main a behavior), and using other types of behavior modification techniques (e.g., rewarding positive behaviors). Behavior modification refers to techniques that assist in teaching new behaviors, that are positive in nature, and techniques to reduce the occurrence of negative behaviors, such as self-injurious or aggressive behaviors. Shaping behavior (using small steps or components of the behavior until they are chained to produce the desired behavior), reinforcing or rewarding positive behaviors, and ignoring or not rewarding negative behaviors are some principles that are key tenets of behavior modification.

ABA specialists have significant expertise in behavior modification techniques. For example, ABA specialists may apply a functional analysis of behavior to determine a plan to change a child's behavior. To do this the professional will observe the child's behaviors to understand what triggers the behavior and what factors in the child's environment reward or help the child to initiate or maintain the behavior. The ABA specialist designs plans to reward desired behaviors and ignore or remove reinforcement from those behaviors that are not positive for the child. The ABA specialist also carefully gathers data to record change in the target behavior or the behavior that the intervention is designed to change. Decisions about whether a child's behavior has changed are based on data, typically using behavior observations to denote change in the frequency of desired behaviors (e.g., increase in frequency) and decrease in negative or undesired behaviors (e.g., decrease in the frequency of self-harm behaviors or other types of negative behaviors).

Medications

Many different medications have been used to treat children with ASD. Because of the intense emotional burden experienced by the parents, they may be very eager for any type of cure. They should be referred to experts in the field, such as developmental pediatricians (pediatricians that have significant expertise in the treatment of developmental disabilities, like ASD), or child psychiatrists with expertise in the treatment of ASD for any type of medication evaluation. Children with severe symptoms may be treated with psychotropic or other medications. Psychotropic medications impact cognitive functioning (thinking), emotional functioning, and behavior. Some of these types of medications can have significant side effects. Administration of many other types of medications has been documented (including stimulants, sleep medications, etc.; Murray et al., 2014). Medical management is very complex and individualized and is beyond the scope of this chapter.

Psychosocial and Emotional Functioning

There is a high degree of parent stress and parents have a significant amount of "burden" or caregiver burden when caring for their child with ASD (Kogan et al., 2009). The burden typically is consistent with the degree of impairment that the child is experiencing. Children with ASD can have different types of emotional and behavioral problems (Maskey, Warnell, Parr, Le Couteur, & McConachie, 2013). Children can display aggression, as well as problems with sleep and eating. In terms of eating behaviors, children can be quite "picky," liking only certain food textures or eating only certain types of foods (children may eat only a very limited range of foods). Children can be very active or inactive, with differences in activity level that are very different from what might be considered "normal" for children. Children with ASD may be less sensitive to pain, and have difficulty letting adults know what they are experiencing pain. When feeling frustrated, which may be exacerbated by low abilities to communicate using language, children with ASD may be likely to engage in self-injurious behaviors. Two examples of self-injurious behaviors include head-banging and hand-biting. The impact of self-injurious behaviors can be especially concerning if the child has a diminished pain response, because he or she might not feel pain when engaging in self-injurious behavior. Children can also have unique sensory preferences, such as preferences for flashing lights and spinning objects, and they may engage in stereotypies. When these sensory preferences are repeated for self-stimulation, these sensory behaviors are the types of repetitive behaviors (stereotypies) which can be hallmark features when making a diagnosis of ASD. Children with ASD can experience a great deal of anxiety, in social situations and when their routines change.

Children with ASD often experience significant deficits in social skills and have great difficulties in making friends (see Petrina, Carter, & Stephenson, 2014 for a review). They may not make "good eye contact" and have difficulty looking another person "in the eye." They may have difficulty using the words "you" and "I" in social conversations. If the child is "echoing" parts of what the other children are saying this can be frustrating to the child's peers. The other children, who are interacting with the child with ASD, may feel that the child is not able to have a conversation with or play with them. Children with ASD may have difficulty taking turns in conversations and talking about others' interests or taking others' perspectives, making social interactions between them and their peers very awkward. Children with ASD may have few friends and feel lonely. Many of the children can identify what friendships are and understand that they have difficulty socially and have few friends. Children with ASD may be satisfied with the friends they have, however. Petrina et al. (2014) have called for more research to determine satisfaction with existing friendships for children who have ASD. It is important to note that a lack of social bonds and social development is a key factor that is related to emotional and behavioral difficulties as children age, and thus a lack of social connection can have long-term implications for a child's social development.

Interventions

Early diagnosis or diagnosing ASD at young ages is critical, given that there is evidence that early intervention with very young children can be particularly effective in improving social and emotional functioning (Mandell, Novak, & Zubritsky, 2005). Early and intensive intervention with preschool-age children who have ASD may be particularly effective in improving their functioning (Eikeseth, Klintwall, Jahr, & Karlsson, 2012). These interventions typically involve using behavior modification techniques, which often are administered by Applied Behavior Analysis or ABA specialists. Significant parent involvement in behavior change plans and in practicing with the child often is necessary. The principles of early and intensive intervention employed by Eikeseth et al. were based on the principles of applied behavior analysis (ABA).

ABA techniques were used by Ivar Lovaas (2003), who is the father of the "UCLA model." This model involves ABA, where children's social skills are developed in applied settings (i.e., in schools and other real-world settings) using behavior modification techniques. There is continuous evaluation of the effectiveness of the intervention techniques. The Lovaas Institute has details about training young children with ASD, typically between the ages of 2 through 8, using ABA (see http://www.lovaas.com/ accessed on December 28, 2015). The UCLA model emphasizes the use of language for social communication and reduction in repetitive or self-stimulatory behaviors. Repetitive and negative behaviors are redirected toward developmentally appropriate positive behaviors (these are appropriate behaviors given the child's age range). These appropriate behaviors are desired, prosocial behavioral alternatives. Positive behaviors are reinforced with rewards the child likes. If a child is not able to exhibit appropriate behaviors for his or her age range, then positive behaviors that the child can perform will be taught. Maladaptive or negative behaviors, such as yelling at one's mother, do not receive reinforcement (e.g., ignoring negative behaviors). Discrete trails are used to teach simple skills progressing to more complex positive behaviors (Volkmar et al., 2014). Discrete trial training occurs when a behavior is broken down into small steps and the progression of small steps are chained together until the child learns the behavior (Bogin, Sullivan, Rogers, & Stabel, 2010). In addition to appropriate social interactions, children learn imitation, play, and how to follow instructions. Lovaas (2003) provided detailed information about behavioral techniques in his book entitled, "Teaching Individuals with Developmental Delays: Basic Intervention Techniques."

In their study, Eikeseth et al. (2012) assigned children with ASD to an intensive behavioral intervention or a treatment as usual group, which was the comparison group. Children ranged in age from 2 through 7 years (mean or average age was about 4 years). Those children assigned to the "treatment" group participated in ABA interventions, which were delivered by teachers. The ABA interventions were adapted from the UCLA Method (Lovaas, 2003). As mentioned, behaviorally based treatments, such as ABA, involve use of reinforcement of positive behaviors to increase their frequency, and ignoring and a lack of reinforcement for negative behaviors in order to reduce their frequency. Children in the ABA interventions group received an average of 23 h of intervention per week (range 15–37 h). These interventions involved implementation of ABA techniques using individualized programs for children. Use of language for social communication was reinforced and repetitive or self-stimulatory behaviors were redirected toward other positive behaviors. Children were reinforced for small steps that slowly shaped their behavior toward a goal behavior. These small steps, as the behavior is "shaped" to more closely resemble the desired or target behavior are termed successive approximations. Discrete trial training, which was defined earlier in this chapter, was used. Rewards or reinforcers for adaptive behaviors were selected based on the child's unique preferences or personal "likes." Social interaction was built around children's preferred activities and cooperative social interactions and play with peers were emphasized. Detailed behavioral plans, with continuous evaluation, and parent involvement were emphasized. Parents learned how to teach similar behaviors to those taught by teachers at home.

Children in the comparison group (who received treatment as usual in the community) received a variety of interventions that focused on learning appropriate play behaviors, self-help skills, social skills, and improving social communication (Eikeseth et al., 2012). Children in the comparison group could also receive sensory integration training involving rocking, swinging, messaging, etc. Children's progress in adaptive functioning was measured a year later and children in the treatment group showed significantly higher levels of adaptive behavior than those in the comparison group (Eikeseth et al.). Children in the treatment group also showed gains in reducing maladaptive behaviors compared to those in the comparison group. These findings are important, because school staff delivered the interventions and they had not received special training. Thus, study results provided support for the idea that behavioral intervention, adapted from the Lovaas (2003) method could be delivered by school staff in the "real world" and have a positive impact on improving the functioning of young children with ASD.

Aduen, Rich, Sanchez, O'Brien, and Alvord (2014) examined a manualized intervention to improve social skills and resiliency for children with ASD. This intervention was delivered using a treatment manual, which outlined interventions and how to deliver interventions to children. Having a manualized intervention allows for consistency in administration and the degree to which the intervention was delivered as planned can be evaluated. This can be advantageous, because leaders (instructors) follow the same plan and administer the same interventions in the same ways. If an intervention is delivered using a manual, then one can also measure the degree to which the leaders followed the manual when delivering the intervention. Leaders can complete surveys showing how they followed the steps in the manual or leaders can be videotaped and review of videotapes can show how closely that leaders were following the training outlined in the manual.

The intervention used by Aduen et al. (2014) was called the Resilience Builder Program. Children participating in this intervention were children between the ages of 7 and 12 years (average age about 10 years old). There were 12 boys and 5 girls and 14 of the participants were Caucasian. The youth participating in this program

Table 6.1 Lessons used in the Resilience Builder Program for children with ASD

Session	Components of the session
1	*Introduction*: Meet others and learn the purpose of the intervention
2	*Resilience*—Learn the concept of resilience and how to be proactive rather than reactive in social interactions. Teaching children to be flexible was emphasized
3	*Personal space*—Understand the distance needed between individuals when they interact. Learn about speed of speech and movement in social situations
4	*Leadership*—How to be a good leader—being flexible, listening to and meeting others' needs, being a role model, etc.
5	*Reading verbal and nonverbal behaviors*—Read children's cues through watching videos and role-play interventions. Flexibility in responding to other children's responses was emphasized
6	*Initiating and maintaining conversations*—How to make eye contact and initiate and maintain conversations. Learn about conversation "busters" that tend to end conversations with others
7	*Good sportsmanship*—Learn how to complement others, control frustration, and play fair when the demands of the game (interaction) change
8	*Optimistic thinking*—Difference between optimistic and pessimistic thinking defined. Learn how to change maladaptive thinking to more positive thinking
9	*Problem-solving*—Learn adaptive and flexible ideas for solving problems. Opportunities to practice problem-solving to improve mental flexibility
10	*Stress management*—Learn stress management and relaxation skills. Development of coping plans is reviewed
11	*Generalization training*—Practice skills on a field trip, such as going bowling together
12	*Perspective-taking*—Learn about empathy and how to understand how others feel in different situations

were considered high functioning and were not exhibiting severe delays in communication, intellectual functioning, and other behaviors associated with the diagnosis of ASD. The Resilience Builder Program consisted of 12 sessions, each lasting 1 h. Aduen et al. used cognitive behavioral techniques to improve social skills and emotion regulation. The sessions addressed several skills, which are presented in Table 6.1.

Aduen et al. (2014) used a variety of measurement tools to examine child progress after participating in their intervention. Their findings indicated that parents reported improvement in child social engagement (social interactions with others) after their children had participated in the program. Children reported that they had better control of their emotions and were using less negative emotions when they were interacting with others. Teachers also completed surveys to assess change in child functioning. Teachers' responses did not indicate significant changes in child functioning. Also, family functioning remained unchanged. Aduen et al. reported that study findings indicated that the program yielded some success, but that improvements were not consistent for teachers, parents, and children. Because results were not consistent for all three groups, in terms of child improvement, Aduen et al. recommended future research to examine the effectiveness of their program. Also, family functioning did not improve, which is another reason they recommended that more research would be needed to determine whether the program was effective. Developing additional lessons to address negative behaviors and reduce repetitive behaviors may strengthen the intervention. Moreover, there was only one session devoted to generalizing what the children learned to other similar types of social situations. Adding sessions to allow children to practice their new skills in different settings or having a coach to ensure that they are practicing what they had learned at home and in the community may increase the impact of the Resilience Builders' lessons.

Roles for Health Educators

Health educators can play a role in referring children for evaluation. Mental health clinicians can make diagnoses. It is important to remember to use multiple measures, parent interview, and observations to gather diagnostic information. After a formal diagnosis is obtained, health educators may be instrumental in the delivery of interventions to improve children's social skills, reduce repetitive behaviors, improve abilities to manage tasks of daily living, and improve emotion regulation. Health educators may want to participate in ABA training to learn key principles of behavior modification, in order to design state of the art interventions. Health educators can improve their training in ABA methods so that they can help in administering or developing behavior plans to improve social and emotional functioning of children with ASD. All of the aforementioned areas are critical areas for improving the lives of children with ASD. Working with school staff and teachers to develop Individual Education Programs will improve school support.

Case Study

Andrew is an 8-year-old child who has been diagnosed with ASD. He has very loving parents who are very involved in his life. He has a 12-year-old sister, who is developing normally. There was not any history of social difficulties or emotional problems in his family according to his parents. Both of his parents describe themselves as being "loners" in terms of preferring their "alone time" to engaging in interactions with large groups of people. There is not a history of mental illness on either Andrew's mother's or fathers' side of the family. Andrew is considered to be high functioning. He is reading and completing math problems at the same level as his peers in the classroom. His social skills are much less well developed than those of peers in his classroom. Moreover, his social use of speech, to communicate with peers, is delayed. Andrew has an Individual Education Program to address his special needs in the school setting. In addition, having an Individual Education Program ensures that his academic progress will be reviewed and updated regularly.

Andrew has been receiving special services since he received a diagnosis of ASD at 3 years of age. He has received behaviorally oriented services to reduce his stereotypical behavior, which was spinning objects and repetitive hand-flapping. Occasionally, he still engages in these behaviors when he is upset. Andrew has received special training, in one-on-one sessions, to improve his eye contact and ability to "pass the ball" in conversations and take turns when speaking with others. Andrew has learned to think about how other children are feeling through lessons stressing perspective-taking with his therapist. He responds very well to rewards. It is important to develop a reward chart focused on things Andrew likes, which include time to review his maps (he has quite a large collection) and extra time to play games on his computer at home or games on a computer in the computer room at his school.

Andrew can become upset when his routine changes. For example, he can become upset when there is a substitute teacher in his classroom or the "order" of his typical classroom schedule changes, such as when there is a special field trip or an assembly. Andrew has learned special breathing techniques to calm down and to ask his teacher for some time at his desk so he can adjust to changes in routine. Andrew responds very well to visual reminders, such as lists, that allow him to understand when there will be changes in his daily routine. The list typically has highlighted changes to the order of activities in his usual routine, when he has a schedule change. Andrew works with his school counselor and his therapist to assist him with practicing social skills and emotion regulation skills. This extra practice and coaching has helped Andrew by reinforcing the social skills he learned as a preschooler and helping him learn new skills to interact with children at his school. Andrew can have trouble understanding social interactions. His counselor at school and his therapist communicate regularly to develop interventions to help him in social situations with peers. The school counselor has an excellent relationship with the classroom teacher and can help in the classroom on an as-needed basis should difficulties arise.

Andrew is enrolled in boy scouts. His scout master knows about his diagnosis and can reach his therapist should difficulties arise. Andrew has a peer buddy at meetings. His buddy helps him when he has difficulty interacting with other boys or goes to find the leader of his scout group, who helps Andrew with social situations he is having difficulty understanding. Andrew's peer buddy and his scout group leader help him to initiate conversations, remind him to make eye contact with peers, and help him complete projects if he is falling behind. When needed, his father comes to group meetings with Andrew to help him complete projects. Andrew is very proud of his merit badges, and he enjoys going camping with his father and the rest of his peers. Andrew's peers have a good understanding of his social delays. They understand that he can have difficulty calming down when routines change or he does not understand what is happening in social interactions. Andrew's therapist had attended a meeting with his peers and explained some of Andrew's challenges to them, which put many of the boys at ease about working with Andrew.

Andrew is doing very well, but probably will need continued support to manage emotional reactions to change, and to assist him in interacting with peers, especially in situations that are "new" for Andrew (e.g., situations that are new or different from his usual routine). His teachers and leaders of the after-school programs he is involved in will need special guidance and support to work with Andrew. His school counselor and therapist plan to remain involved throughout the elementary school years. His educational attainment remains good, and his academic progress, as well as his social and emotional development, will be assessed yearly or more frequently if this is needed. A larger scale evaluation will be conducted every 3 years as part of his Individual Education Programming. Additional supports may be needed in the middle and high school years, as social demands and situations with peers increase in complexity. In the long-term, in high school, planning for his early adult years will be important so that he can attain to his highest potential in the least restrictive environment.

Summary

In this chapter, diagnosis of ASD and ideas for assessment and treatment were reviewed. A lack of social interaction and social communication are hallmark features of ASD. Therefore, intervention programs typically must address skills deficits in these areas. Children with ASD may exhibit repetitive, restrictive patterns of behavior. They may experience difficulty transitioning to different activities, especially when there are changes in their usual routine. They may have difficulty completing work "on demand" or when asked to complete a task or assignment. In addition, a fairly high number of children with ASD experience delays in intellectual functioning. Interventions for children with ASD often involve ABA. This is a behavioral approach where a functional analysis of behavior is used to determine an intervention plan for different types of behaviors that need to change or be modified. Careful data collection, typically based on behavior observations, is used to assess change. Future research to identify interventions that result in significant improvement in social skills and reduction in negative behaviors will continue to improve the future of children who have ASD.

Exercises/Review Questions

1. Caregivers or parents can become very stressed upon hearing that their child has been diagnosed with ASD. How would you explain this diagnosis to them?
2. What are stereotypies?
3. How would you explain ASD to a classroom of young elementary school-age children who were having difficulty interacting with and understanding the repetitive behaviors of a peer with ASD?
4. What steps would you use to teach a boy with ASD, who is in kindergarten, and who is having trouble sharing toys with other children in the classroom? Please break your teaching into small steps with rewards for approximations or positive movements toward the desired sharing behavior you have defined. Then, discuss a plan for observing the child and collecting data to determine the child's progress in improving abilities to share with peers.

5. Describe how you might observe and conduct a functional analysis of behavior (observing triggers for a behavior, the consequences of a behavior, and rewards for a behavior) for a child with an ASD who has a problem with biting his hands when he has to transition between activities during the school day.
6. If you developed a school-based program for first- or second-grade children with ASD what would be key components of your program to improve their communication with other children?

Key Concepts

Autism Spectrum Disorder (ASD)
Severity levels for children with ASD
Stereotypies
Echolalia
Narrow range of interests
DISCO
M-CHAT
CARS
Behavior modification
Shaping
Reinforcement
ABA training
UCLA model
Discrete trial training
Resilience Builder Program

References

Aduen, P. A., Rich, B. A., Sanchez, L., O'Brien, K., & Alvord, M. K. (2014). Resilience Builder Program therapy addresses core social deficits and emotion dysregulation in youth with high-functioning autism spectrum disorder. *Journal of Psychological Abnormalities in Children, 3*(2), 118–128. doi:10.4172/2329-9525.1000118.

American Psychiatric Association. (2013). *Diagnostic and statistical manual of mental disorders* (5th ed.). Washington, DC: Author.

Becerra, T. A., von Ehrenstein, O. S., Heck, J. E., Olsen, J., Arah, O. A., Jeste, S. S., … Ritz, B. (2014). Autism spectrum disorders and race, ethnicity, and nativity: A population-based study. *Pediatrics, 134*, e63–e71. doi: 10.1542/peds.2013-3928.

Bogin, J., Sullivan, L., Rogers, S., & Stabel, A. (2010). *Steps for implementation: Discrete trial training*. Sacramento, CA: The National Professional Development Center on Autism Spectrum Disorders, The M.I.N.D. Institute, The University of California at Davis School of Medicine. Retrieved December 28, 2015, from http://csesa.fpg.unc.edu/sites/csesa.fpg.unc.edu/files/ebp-briefs/DTT_Steps_0.pdf.

Carrington, S. J., Kent, R. G., Maljaars, J., Le Couteur, A., Gould, J., Wing, L., … Leekam, S. R. (2014). DSM-V autism spectrum disorder: In search of essential behaviors for diagnosis. *Research in Autism Spectrum Disorders, 8*(6), 701–715. doi: 10.1016/j.rasd.2014.03.017.

Carrington, S., Leekam, S., Kent, R., Maljaars, J., Gould, J., Wing, L., ... Noens, I. (2015). Signposting for diagnosis of autism spectrum disorder using the Diagnostic Interview for Social and Communication Disorders (DISCO). *Research in Autism Spectrum Disorders, 9*, 45–52.

Cunningham, A. B., & Schreibman, L. (2008). Stereotypy in autism: The importance of function. *Research in Autism Spectrum Disorders, 2*(3), 469–479.

Eikeseth, S., Klintwall, L., Jahr, E., & Karlsson, P. (2012). Outcome for children with autism receiving early and intensive behavioral intervention in mainstream preschool and kindergarten setting. *Research in Autism Spectrum Disorders, 6*, 829–835. doi:10.1016/j.rasd.2011.09.002.

Gotham, K., Bishop, S. L., Hus, V., Huerta, M., Lund, S., Buja, A., ... Lord, C. (2013). Exploring the relationship between anxiety and insistence on sameness in autism spectrum disorders. *Autism Research, 6*(1), 33–41.

Grossi, D., Marcone, R., Cinquegrana, T., & Gallucci, M. (2013). On the differential nature of induced and incidental echolalia in autism. *Journal of Intellectual Disability Research, 57*(10), 903–912.

Herlihy, L. E., Brooks, B., Dumont-Mathieu, T., Barton, M. L., Fein, D., Chen, C. M., & Robins, D. L. (2014). Standardized screening facilitates timely diagnosis of autism spectrum disorders in a diverse sample of low-risk toddlers. *Journal of Developmental and Behavioral Pediatrics, 35*(2), 85–92.

Kogan, M. D., Blumberg, S. J., Schieve, L. A., Boyle, C. A., Perrin, J. M., Ghandour, R. M., ... van Dyck, P. C. (2009). Prevalence of parent-reported diagnosis of autism spectrum disorder among children in the U.S. 2007. *Pediatrics, 124*(4), 1395–1403. doi: 10.1542/peds.2009-1522.

Kulage, K. M., Smaldone, A. M., & Cohn, E. G. (2014). How will DSM-5 affect autism diagnosis? A systematic literature review and meta-analysis. *Journal of Autism and Developmental Disorders, 44*(8), 1918–1932. doi:10.1007/s10803-014-2065-2.

Lidstone, J., Uljarević, M., Sullivan, J., Rodgers, J., McConachie, H., Freeston, M., ... Leekam, S. (2014). Relations among restricted and repetitive behaviors, anxiety and sensory features in children with autism spectrum disorders. *Research in Autism Spectrum Disorders, 8*(2), 82–92. doi: 10.1016/j.rasd.2013.10.001.

Lovaas, O. I. (2003). *Teaching individuals with developmental delays: Basic intervention techniques.* Austin, TX: PRO-ED.

Mandell, D. S., Novak, M. M., & Zubritsky, C. D. (2005). Factors associated with age of diagnosis among children with autism spectrum disorders. *Pediatrics, 116*(6), 1480–1486. doi:10.1542/peds.2005-0185.

Maskey, M., Warnell, F., Parr, J. R., Le Couteur, A., & McConachie, H. (2013). Emotional and behavioural problems in children with autism spectrum disorder. *Journal of Autism and Developmental Disorders, 43*(4), 851–859.

Murray, M. L., Hsia, Y., Glaser, K., Simonoff, E., Murphy, D. G., Asherson, P. J., ... Wong, I. C. (2014). Pharmacological treatments prescribed to people with autism spectrum disorder (ASD) in primary health care. *Psychopharmacology, 231*(6), 1011–1021.

Petrina, N., Carter, M., & Stephenson, J. (2014). The nature of friendship in children with autism spectrum disorders: A systematic review. *Research in Autism Spectrum Disorders, 8*, 111–126.

Robins, D. L., Casagrande, K., Barton, M., Chen, C.-M. A., Durmont-Mathieu, T., & Fein, D. (2014). Validation of the Modified Checklist for Autism in Toddlers, Revised with Follow-Up (M-CHAT-R/F). *Pediatrics, 133*(1), 37–45.

Robins, D. L., Fein, D., & Barton, M. (1999). The Modified Checklist for Autism in Toddlers (M-CHAT). Authors.

Robins, D. L., Fein, D., & Barton, M. (2009). The Modified Checklist for Autism in Toddlers, Revised (M-CHAT-R). Authors. Retrieved from https://m-chat.org/print.php.

Schopler, E., Reichler, R. J., DeVellis, R. F., & Daly, K. (1980). Toward objective classification of childhood autism: Childhood Autism Rating Scale (CARS). *Journal of Autism and Developmental Disorders, 10*(1), 91–103. doi:10.1007/BF02408436.

Schopler, E., Van Bourgondien, M. E., Wellman, G. J., & Love, S. R. (2010). *Child autism rating scale ™* (2nd ed.). Torrance, CA: Western Psychological Services (WPS).

Volkmar, F., Siegel, M., Woodbury-Smith, M., King, B., McCracken, J., & State, M. (2014). Practice parameter for the assessment and treatment of children and adolescents with autism spectrum disorder. *Journal of the American Academy of Child & Adolescent Psychiatry, 53*(2), 237–257.

Chapter 7
Anxiety

Diagnosis

Anxiety is a broad and "diffuse" concept, making it difficult to define (Vasey, Bosmans, & Ollendick, 2014). There are many definitions of anxiety. For example, Fonseca and Perrin (2011) defined anxiety as, "…a set of emotional reactions arising from the anticipation of a real or imagined threat to the self" (p. 25). Fonseca and Perrin differentiated anxiety from fear, in that fear is a reaction to a distinguishable stimulus, whereas anxiety may be a less specific reaction to a diffuse array of stimuli. Experts have proposed that anxiety is the most common form of mental health disorder in children (e.g., Vasey et al., 2014). Fonesca and Perrin discussed that, with the exception of Generalized Anxiety Disorder (GAD; formerly Overanxious Disorder of Childhood) and Separation Anxiety Disorder (SAD), most diagnoses involving anxiety are the same (i.e., involve the same types of symptoms) for children and adults.

There are several systems for classifying anxiety; however, the most common is to use the *Diagnostic and Statistical Manual of Mental Disorders* (American Psychiatric Association, 2013). In DSM-5, anxiety is defined as, "… the anticipation of a future threat" (p. 189). Feelings of anxiety must be persistent and strong enough to interfere with the child's daily functioning and ability to perform daily tasks for a significant period of time. The onset of symptoms often occurs around 6 years of age (Merikangas et al., 2010). Children who are anxious may be overly conforming to social norms or rules. They may be worried about their performance at school or at sports, making them appear to be "perfectionists" (American Psychiatric Association, 2013).

There are many anxiety disorders described in the DSM-5, such as Post-Traumatic Stress Disorder, SAD, GAD, and Social Phobia (see Vasey et al., 2014 or the DSM-5, American Psychiatric Association, 2013 for a review). There is some "overlap" in symptoms among the different anxiety disorders in children—such that similar symptoms are displayed across disorders (Copeland, Angold, Shanahan, &

© Springer International Publishing Switzerland 2016
L. Nabors, *Medical and Mental Health During Childhood*, Springer
Series on Child and Family Studies, DOI 10.1007/978-3-319-31117-3_7

Costello, 2014). Nonetheless, there is enough difference among the diagnoses to use separate diagnostic categories for the many types of anxiety disorders. Seven anxiety disorders will be defined on in the next section of this chapter: SAD, GAD, Social Anxiety Disorder, Selective Mutism, Obsessive-Compulsive Disorder, School Phobia, and Specific Phobia.

Separation Anxiety Disorder. Separation anxiety is described as being, "fearful or anxious about separation from attachment figures to a degree that is developmentally inappropriate" (American Psychiatric Association, 2013, p. 189). Children with separation anxiety can experience worry about the loss or separation from an attachment figure, to the extent that they experience nightmares and physiological symptoms (e.g., tremor, upset stomach, rapid breathing rate). Separation anxiety typically is present for at least 4 weeks in children who are diagnosed with this disorder.

Generalized Anxiety Disorder. This disorder is defined as, "…excessive anxiety and worry…about a number of events or activities" (American Psychiatric Association, 2013, p. 222). The worry that the child experiences is "out of proportion" or very high given the likelihood that the event that is being worried about will actually occur. Children with GAD may worry about their competence or performance at school or for sports/activities. Children can also worry about catastrophic events, such as floods or earthquakes (American Psychiatric Association, 2013). Children with significant anxiety may be perfectionists. Their work may need to be perfect or their performance perfect, or they will start over on a current project or performance. They may be receiving a lot of reassurance from others, which can paradoxically increase their worries (because they are being reaffirmed by parental attention).

Social Anxiety Disorder. This disorder is characterized by fear and avoidance of social situations. Children with social anxiety disorder may avoid social situations, worry about negative evaluations by others, be self-conscious, and have a limited number of friends. These children may have appropriate social skills (Rapee, 2012).

Selective Mutism. This disorder is defined as failure to speak in social situations, where there is an expectation that individuals will speak with others (American Psychiatric Association, 2013). Children with Selective Mutism may be very shy and experience fear in social situations. Typically, the child has no problems with his or her speaking abilities and does not have a communication disorder. The child most often speaks with his or her immediate family, but may not speak with grandparents or other family members. This can be very distressing for the family. Parents of children with selective mutism may also experience social inhibition or be inhibited. They can also be controlling, and overly controlling of the child.

Obsessive-Compulsive Disorder. This disorder is characterized by obsessions and/or compulsions or compulsive behavior (Abramowitz, Taylor, & McKay, 2009). Obsessions are repetitive, intrusive thoughts. Compulsive behaviors are repetitive behaviors that one feels compelled to perform. Compulsive behaviors are often performed in response to obsessive thinking, typically in a rigid, ritualistic fashion. The compulsions can be a kind of undoing, where the individual performs a behavior to relieve stress related to experiencing obsessive thoughts. The individual may believe that performing the ritualistic behavior can help him or her ward off anxiety-provoking events. The compulsive behavior can reinforce the anxious thinking—in terms of obsessive worry—because performing the ritual reinforces the belief or the anxiety related to the obsessive thought. Obsessions can center on fear of causing harm. Compulsions then can become checking compulsions to ensure safety. Obsessions focusing on contamination (e.g., worry about germs) can be accompanied by compulsive handwashing rituals.

School Phobia. This disorder is often termed school refusal (Kahn, Nursten, & Carroll, 1981; Maynard et al., 2015). Children with school refusal or school phobia refuse to go to school. Children with School Phobia may experience anxiety—to the level of panic—over needing to go to school. They may want to remain at home. They may have many absences. Unlike children who may be truant for conduct problems, children with school refusal often want to go to school, but feel that they cannot do so. Thus, school phobia is "…an emotional problem, based on acute anxiety at the thought of leaving home" (p. 5, Kahn et al., 1981).

Specific Phobia. This is an excessive and persistent fear of a specific stimuli or event (American Psychiatric Association, 2013; Ollendick et al., 2015). The feared stimuli or event can be of animals; natural events in the environment (e.g., thunder); blood, injection, or injury; a situation (e.g., giving a speech), or be another type of fear of a different stimuli or event, which is classified as having an "other" type of phobia. Children with fears of specific stimuli generally benefit from gradual exposure to the feared stimuli. This allows them to confront and work through their fear of the object, as their fear is excessive and unrealistic (Ollendick et al., 2015).

Prevalence of Anxiety in Children

Approximately 5–10 % of children experience an anxiety disorder (Cobham, 2012; Drake & Ginsburg, 2012; March, Spence, & Donovan, 2009). Rates of anxiety for children differ from 2.8 % to over 30 % across studies (Copeland et al., 2014; Costello, Egger, & Angold, 2005; Reynolds, Wilson, Austin, & Hooper, 2012). Results of other national studies show that as many as one in eight children and adolescents experience some form of anxiety (Merikangas et al., 2010). Uncertainty about the definition or description of anxiety disorders in children may influence the differing prevalence rates across studies (Costello et al., 2005). Symptoms of anxiety in children are similar across cultures (Holly, Little, Pina, & Caterino, 2015; Vasey et al., 2014). Rates of anxiety may increase in the adolescent years (Copeland et al., 2014). Rates may increase in adolescence, perhaps because in adolescence the expression of anxiety symptoms "look" much more like adult symptoms and adolescents are more able to describe anxiety symptoms than younger children.

As might be expected, the prevalence of the different types of anxiety disorders varies across studies. According to the DSM-5 (American Psychiatric Association, 2013), SAD occurs in about 4 % of children. It is the most prevalent mental health problem in children aged 7 years and younger (Santucci & Ehrenreich-May, 2013). GAD appears to be less common among children (less than 1 %). Selective mutism occurs in .03–1 % of children (American Psychiatric Association, 2013). The prevalence of obsessive compulsive disorder is between 0.5 and 3 % (Torp et al., 2015). Specific phobias are present in as many as, "…5 % of children in community samples" (p. 2, Ollendick et al., 2015).

There are fairly clear gender differences across studies. Girls are more likely to be diagnosed with anxiety than boys, and this is true for most types of anxiety disorders (American Psychiatric Association, 2013; Copeland et al., 2014; Costello et al., 2005). Girls may be up to two times more likely to be diagnosed with an anxiety disorder compared to boys (Rapee, 2012).

Information about differences between ethnic or racial groups is less clear. For example, Holly et al. (2015) examined anxiety in 702 children who were white or Hispanic. After adjusting the survey for cultural differences in responses to questions, their findings indicated that anxiety symptoms were at an equal level for boys who were white, boys who were Hispanic, and girls who were Hispanic. About 6–7 % of the children in these groups (boys who were white and who were Hispanic and girls who were Hispanic) were experiencing anxiety. Girls who were white were experiencing more symptoms of anxiety; about 9 % of girls who were white were reporting symptoms of anxiety.

Genetic and Environmental Influences. Anxiety disorders have a genetic component and "run in families." There is support from studies with twins and of parents with anxiety to support the heritable nature of anxiety disorders (Drake & Ginsburg, 2012). However, the environment, chiefly parental influences, can play a role in the development of anxiety for children. Drake and Ginsburg (2012) reviewed parental influences on child anxiety and noted several important findings from the literature. For example, parents who are unpredictable and foster an insecure attachment with the child increase anxiety symptoms, such as hypervigilance, in children. In addition, parents who are very controlling and overinvolved in their children's lives may facilitate the development of anxiety in children, because children do not get to practice working through and achieving success in challenging situations (Drake & Ginsburg). Another reason children may learn to exhibit anxiety is that they are modeling or copying parental coping strategies and thought processes, including anxious ones (Hudson et al., 2014). Parents also may reinforce children's anxiety by helping them avoid feared stimuli or allowing them, albeit inadvertently, to be very worried and avoid situations that make them worried. This parental accommodation, which can also extend to other family members, may actually heighten the child's anxiety symptoms and feelings of worry (Norman, Silverman, & Lebowitz, 2015).

Impact for Children

In this chapter, the focus will be on a general discussion of how anxiety impacts children. Ideas will be cross-cutting, in that they will assist health professionals in working with children who experience anxiety, irrespective of the specific type of anxiety disorder with which they are diagnosed. The goal will be to assist health educators and professionals in being able to identify, refer, and provide coping strategies to help children who are experiencing anxiety. There are specific cognitive-behavioral treatments that work "better" or were specifically designed for different types of anxiety disorders; but, addressing all of the specific treatments is beyond the scope of this chapter. On the other hand, there are some treatments that work for several disorders, and these general ideas will be reviewed. Developing expertise in the field, through reading, supervised experiences, coursework, and clinical experiences will help the student gain expertise in treating specific anxiety disorders.

Anxiety disorders can co-occur or are comorbid with other mental health conditions. The most common comorbid problem is another anxiety disorder (Fonseca & Perrin, 2011; Reynolds et al., 2012). Another common coexisting problem is having depression (Costello et al., 2005). Indeed, some have categorized depression and anxiety as sharing a common factor—the experience of negative affect or a negative mood state. Depression would involve negative affect and a lack of positive mood. In turn, anxiety would involve negative affect and physiological hyperarousal (Clark & Watson, 1991). Childhood anxiety is also related to other problems, such as lower academic performance, difficulties in peer relationships, and externalizing or "acting out problems" such as disruptive or oppositional behaviors (Costello et al., 2005; Grover, Ginsburg, & Ialongo, 2007). Childhood anxiety symptoms may develop after experiencing a trauma or a significant life stressor, such as loss of a pet or difficulties in the family (American Psychiatric Association, 2013; Grover et al., 2007). Anxiety disorders are likely to recur and/or continue. Grover et al. (2007) found that children with higher levels of anxiety in the first grade had higher levels of anxiety in the seventh grade. In addition, SAD, usually diagnosed in young children, can continue to become social phobia in older children (Costello et al., 2005).

Very young children who are "behaviorally inhibited" may be likely to experience anxiety as they grow and develop. Children with behavioral inhibition may be withdrawn, shy, or anxious in new situations with strangers. They are not "outgoing" in new or unfamiliar situations. Biederman et al. (2001) assessed behavioral inhibition in children between the ages of 2 through 6 years. They found that young children with behavioral inhibition were more likely to experience social anxiety. On the other hand, they concluded that children with behavioral inhibition were less likely to exhibit "acting out" or disruptive types of behavior problems. Similarly, Degnan, Almas, and Fox (2010) proposed that children who experience behavioral inhibitions may be hypervigilant in new situations and withdraw in situations that are worrisome to them, such as social situations. Accordingly, there may be a pattern of anxiety in new situations, related to behavioral inhibition, in the very early years that leads to anxiety symptoms in older children.

Other researchers have proposed that individuals with anxiety have increased levels of high attention to stimuli that are very minor in their threat level. Individuals may orient toward fairly neutral, nonthreatening stimuli, and this may contribute to being hyper-aroused. There is some recent research showing that retraining children's attention to these nonthreatening stimuli, using computer paradigms where a neutral, nonthreatening stimulus is used to retrain the response (anxiety reaction) to the anxiety-provoking stimulus may be a successful treatment (Shechner et al., 2014). How does this occur? Pairing the anxiety-provoking stimulus with a neutral stimulus that is not anxiety provoking, changes the valence of the anxiety-provoking stimulus to be less fear-provoking. This reduces its strength. This occurs with computer training when an anxiety-provoking stimulus is placed in the position of a neutral stimulus on a computer screen. Over repeated trials the child's attention bias is retrained—as attention is "turned away" from the stimuli that were thought to be fear-provoking or anxiety-provoking.

Assessment

When health professionals assess whether children are experiencing anxiety, they need to make a judgment as to whether the anxiety symptoms that the child (or parent) are discussing are at a level considered to be an "extreme" presentation of a fear reaction. Reactions need to be very significant, and interfere with a child's ability to function, as fears are common in children. The fear that the child describes is persistent and strong, so much so that it interferes with the child's ability to function normally or engage in daily activities. Structured interviews are often used in research and/or clinical practice to assess anxiety. One of the most commonly used structured interviews is the Anxiety Disorders Interview Schedule for Children and Parents (ADIS-C/P; Silverman & Albano, 1996). This interview comprises questions that allow the interviewer to move "step by step" through the diagnostic criteria for an anxiety disorder.

Questionnaires are also used to assess or measure children's and caregivers' reports of child anxiety symptoms. There are many questionnaires available. The one selected for discussion in this chapter is the Spence Children's Anxiety Scale (Spence, 1997, 1998). This scale consists of over 40 questions to measure children's levels of anxiety for several symptoms. The questions examine children's opinions of their anxiety for questions measuring several types of anxiety including social anxiety, obsessions and compulsions, general anxiety symptoms and symptoms related to feelings of panic and separation anxiety. This measure is relatively easy for children to complete. There is a parent version as well. These questionnaires are available free of charge. The website can be found at: http://www.scaswebsite.com/1_1_.html (accessed December 30, 2015). Holly, Little, Pina, and Caterino (2015) used the Spence Anxiety scale to examine anxiety in school-age children and found that it was a good instrument for examining symptoms of anxiety in children. The questionnaires have been used to examine how children are progressing when they are receiving treatment for anxiety by a mental health professional or are receiving treatment in an intervention program, such as those discussed later in this chapter. A questionnaire should not be used in isolation or by itself to diagnose anxiety. It is important to have a detailed clinical interview and obtain information from parents and children for several areas of functioning before making a diagnosis. Also, it is advisable for diagnoses to be made by trained mental health professionals.

Disease Management

When working with children and others who experience anxiety, a fundamental principal to remember is that anxiety is not maladaptive. Herbert (2013) stated that anxiety was a normal response, which can be functional. Think of athletes, who often become anxious before a game, and this anxiety can help to spur their best performance (i.e., highest level of skill is produced). Anxiety also exists to protect us against danger, making it a fundamental human response (Herbert, 2013). As a consequence, it is essential to let children and their parents know that feeling anxious is "normal" and that anxious feelings become problematic when they grow disproportionately big, given the situation and the stimulus.

Although the experience of worry, anxiety, and fear has an adaptive base, children who experience anxiety can engage in thinking that is not adaptive for them and has negative outcomes for them (Kendall, 2012). Children may think that things will not turn out positively and that "the worst will happen." Children also may engage in self-blame, thinking of all that they should have done to perform better. This may be related to the tendency for children to worry about their performance or competence when experiencing anxiety (American Psychiatric Association, 2013). They may want their performance to be perfect. Likewise, it may be related to the fact that individuals who experience anxiety often believe that what happens is a result of bad luck, and they feel things are "out of my control." When one feels that "luck" or "fate" controls the outcome of events and situations, the person is said to have an "external locus of control." Children with anxiety disorders may have an external locus of control (Barlow, 2002). This means that they believe things that occur in their lives are largely outside of their control, and this can cause worry and anxiety over the outcomes of the things they do. In these cases, it is important to work with the child to change negative thinking and negative statements to him- or herself and use more positive self-talk ("It's not your fault. Your work does not have to be perfect. You are trying your best and this is great.").

Children can feel that they have to perform perfectly and "get everything just right" and this can be fear-provoking. Kendall (2012) recommended helping the child develop a "coping template." This may involve helping the child reframe his or her tendencies to believe his or her performance has to be perfect or to think that he or she is to blame if things go wrong. The child may also think "things will never turn out right." Teaching the child scripts or sayings that can encourage self-efficacy for going through fears can be a helpful tool. An example script might be, "I can do it. It doesn't have to be perfect." Teaching the child to reframe and reword negative self-talk is an important step in teaching the child a new, more positive coping template. Thus, instead of thinking everything will go wrong, adopting an "it will probably work out and I'll give it a try" attitude or mantra might be a template that would promote and encourage a child to feel positively about facing his or her fears.

There are several systems involved in anxiety including: (1) thinking, (2) feeling, and (3) physical reaction. In terms of thinking, maladaptive thoughts, which are negative in nature, are common. As mentioned, children can think that the worst will happen or that the stimuli causing anxiety are very powerful and cannot be overcome. In terms of feeling, negative mood or "affect" is common. Anxiety can cause a very negative feeling state. The child's physical reaction may involve a state of hyperarousal and this is related to increased breathing, sweating, and shaking (Fonseca & Perrin, 2011). In order to treat the anxiety, the therapist needs to be able to address all three levels—changing negative thinking, replacing negative thinking, and resetting the child's system and helping the child overcome symptoms related to his or her physical reaction to fear (e.g., wanting to run, sweating, and quick and heavy breathing).

One of the most common treatment programs for children with anxiety is the Coping Cat Program (e.g., Kendall, 1994, 2012; Kendall & Hedtke, 2006a, 2006b). Therapists who administer this program begin by assisting a child (and his or her parents) in recognizing the child's anxiety. Therapists help the child recognize anxiety symptoms (maladaptive thinking, physiological distress, avoidance of worrisome or feared events). Therapists teach the children coping strategies, such as muscle relaxation, using positive self-talk, thinking positive things, or "seeing" positive scenes in one's mind (imagery), among other strategies (see Kendall, 2012 for a review). Children learn to recognize which of their facial expressions signal to them that they are experiencing worry or anxiety. Children may learn that their face is becoming tight or that they are frowning, which signals that they are beginning to become upset. Children are taught the acronym "FEAR" (Feelings, Expectations, Actions, and Rewards). In this word, each letter represents a "coping step." For instance, the "F" represents understanding your facial expression and body signs (physiological signs) of anxiety. For "E" children learn to recognize their own expectations (e.g., recognize unrealistic self-talk and expectations for themselves). The "A" stands for action and for "A" children implement the coping strategies they have learned and they try to actively manage their anxiety. For "R" children reward themselves for practicing their coping strategies. This reward can be a small, tangible reward (e.g., piece of candy) or self-praise. The "R" step allows the child to review his or her progress in implementing coping strategies. Kendall et al. (1997) found that use of the Coping Cat strategies and training program resulted in long-term reductions in anxiety and long-term treatment success for children. Kendall's (2012) program is considered a cognitive-behavioral therapy, because the child learns to change his or her negative thoughts and behaviors. Children face their fears and reward positive thinking, which can change their behaviors. And rather than thinking "I will be afraid and I am always going to be scared" children can learn new adaptive thoughts to improve their self-confidence and change thought patterns that promote hyper-arousal and negative affect or mood.

Another key component of treatment for anxiety is graduated exposure to feared stimuli to help the child "go through" his or her anxiety related to the stimuli. A child avoiding an anxiety producing stimuli is accidentally reinforcing the anxiety. The anxiety grows as the child continues to avoid anxiety-provoking stimuli. Consequently, gradual exposure, through modeling, which can occur "live" or "in vivo" or through imaginal rehearsal or video-modeling are interventions to help the child face "anxiety-related" stimuli (Ollendick et al., 2015). The exposure to the feared stimuli can be guided by parents or health professionals who are working with the child in real-world settings. This allows the child to practice working through his or her anxiety with support and guidance. Gradual exposure is often "practiced" with calming self-talk and/or the use of relaxation to help the child to be able to relax and cope with the exposure to the feared stimuli. Another strategy is to gradually expose the child to the feared stimuli while helping him or her "challenge" or dispute faulty cognitions or beliefs. Ollendick et al. (2015) found that brief intervention with children, to teach them about the anxiety cycle, with gradual exposure to the feared stimuli, and the use of challenge statements to overcome negative cognitions was an effective way to treat children with specific phobias (this is a fear of specific things, such as animals, fear of needles).

Medications

Sertraline is an anxiolytic that has been used with children. Serotonin reuptake inhibitors, for example, Fluoxetine, also are prescribed by child psychiatrists and physicians. Medications can be effective when combined with cognitive-behavioral intervention programs. Research is needed to determine further information about how long to use medications, when to stop the medications, and if there are instances when use of medications are contraindicated. Moreover, information is needed about whether it is safe for young children to take medications to treat anxiety (Creswell, Waite, & Cooper, 2014). Developing a relationship with a child psychiatrist or a group of child psychiatrists is beneficial for health educators and others so that they can learn from experts about medication management and childhood anxiety.

Triggers for Anxiety Symptoms

It is important for children to learn physiological triggers for their anxiety symptoms (Albano & Kendall, 2002; Kendall, 2012). Children can learn to recognize what types of "signs or signals in my body" indicate that they are experiencing anxiety. Facial expression can change and learning to recognize facial changes can be one way to recognize precursors or triggers to increasing feelings of anxiety. Other signals may be rapid breathing or tightness in muscles in various parts of the body. Having the child draw an "X" on different body parts on a picture and discuss where he or she "feels his or her worry" may help the child begin to discuss physiological symptoms of anxiety and pinpoint body systems that are involved in his or her anxiety response. If bodily tightness (tensing) or arousal (e.g., accelerated heart rate) is occurring, it can be helpful to teach the child to "reset" his or her system using either deep breathing or muscle relaxation. Young children may have difficulty tensing and relaxing different muscle groups to engage in a full trial of progressive muscle relaxation. Having them tense and relax their entire body, by being a "rock" and then becoming a relaxed "sponge" may be a method for helping children become more relaxed when they begin to feel their body "speed up" or become tense, which enhances anxiety experiences. Another strategy may be to have children squeeze nervous feelings out through making a fist and then waiving "goodbye" to their worries as the anxiety trickles through their fingers.

Psychosocial and Emotional Functioning

Children with anxiety disorders can be "shy" and may be inhibited in terms of expressing emotions (Essau, Conradt, Sasagawa, & Ollendick, 2012). As previously stated, children who are anxious can be "perfectionists," expecting to do things perfectly, resulting in very high expectations for their own performance and being overly concerned with how others evaluate their performance (Essau et al., 2012). Self-esteem may be low for children who experience anxiety (Simon, Dirksen, Bögels, & Bodden, 2012). They may be withdrawn in social situations or lack social skills (Essau et al., 2012; Ollendick, Costa, & Benoit, 2010). They may experience trouble making and maintaining friendships (Drake & Ginsburg, 2012). Children who are anxious can also tend to avoid things that they feel afraid of, and this avoidant coping style can characterize children who have anxiety (Allen, Rapee, & Sanberg, 2008). Interestingly, children who are anxious may experience a higher than average level of stressful events, suggesting that they learn to react to stressors that produce anxiety (Allen et al.). Consequently, it is important to listen to and understand what has happened to cause the child to feel anxiety. There may be many stressors that have been repeated, and through time the child has become over-sensitized to anxiety. Listening and affirming that previous experiences were difficult, but stressing that the child can learn strategies to overcome anxiety, may acknowledge their experiences and help build a foundation for teaching the child strategies to manage fear.

Many children with anxiety may experience difficulties at school, such as poor academic performance (underperforming), and problems with attendance (Drake & Ginsburg, 2012). They tend to follow instructions well in the classroom setting, and therefore they may not experience behavioral difficulties at school. They may tend to hide or mask their symptoms. Because children who are experiencing anxiety "fly under the radar," symptoms of an anxiety disorder can be overlooked. Anxiety disorders can have very serious long-term consequences if untreated. Drake and Ginsburg reported that anxiety disorders that are untreated could result in anxiety, depression, and substance abuse in adulthood.

Interventions for Children with Anxiety

This section of the chapter presents a review of several studies where interventions were used to reduce anxiety symptoms in children. The majority of studies provide treatment to children with several types of anxiety disorders, although some focus on one type of anxiety. The studies chiefly rely on cognitive behavioral therapy (CBT) programs. These types of interventions use techniques to change children's thinking patterns and their behaviors to assist them in reducing feelings of anxiety. CBT interventions also involve exposure to the feared stimulus to decrease the worry associated with this stimulus. There is a heavy educational component to CBT interventions with opportunities for children to practice what they learned during treatment sessions. Group treatments are typically described; however, the strategies used in group treatment can be applied in "one-on-one" sessions with a child and his or her parent. New treatments are still important to explore, especially treatments that will reach children who might not be able to access clinic-based settings to participate in sessions with psychologists or trained mental health therapists. Schools may be optimal settings for developing prevention efforts that will help to prevent anxiety from becoming problematic for children.

March, Spence, and Donovan (2009) implemented an internet-based CBT intervention that was an adaptation of Spence's BRAVE intervention for the treatment of childhood anxiety (Spence, Holmes, March, & Lipp, 2006). The content of the BRAVE intervention was adapted for delivery only through the internet, with colorful illustrations and up-to-date web pages for March et al.'s study. This successful CBT program involved several treatments delivered in child and parent groups (Spence et al., 2006). Children learned to recognize physiological or "body" signs of anxiety. Coping strategies for children included changing negative self-talk and learning new positive thoughts to replace "maladaptive thinking." Slow gradual exposure to feared stimuli was recommended. Consequently, confronting anxiety-provoking stimuli and going through the physiological arousal was proposed to reduce the anxiety associated with the feared stimuli. The children also learned problem-solving, relaxation, imagery, breathing, and muscle relaxation. The child would reward him or herself for "brave" behavior (e.g., coping with anxiety). Children participated in 10, 60-min sessions with booster sessions after the program was completed. In their groups, parents learned about their child's anxiety and learned all the strategies that their children were learning in "child" groups (Spence et al., 2006).

March et al. (2009) found that child anxiety decreased, according to child and parent report. Children had "fewer" anxiety diagnoses after participating in treatment. For the internet program children in the intervention were compared to children in a control group who were going to receive treatment later on, after the treatment group had finished participating in the program. This is commonly referred to as a "wait-list" control group. March et al. (2009) reported that the internet intervention was successful and could offer a cost-savings in terms of therapist effort. Also, internet-based interventions are a good way to reach children who might otherwise not receive treatment as many children with anxiety are not enrolled in clinic-based treatment (Cobham, 2012).

Santucci and Ehrenreich-May (2013) conducted a 7-day camp intervention for girls with SAD. The intervention was built upon CBT interventions and relied on exposure to "separation" in the supportive camp environment with peers experiencing the same issues. Girls between the ages of 7 and 12 years were participants and diagnoses were made by clinicians using the Anxiety Disorders Interview Schedule for Children and Parents (ADIS-C/P; Silverman & Albano, 1996). SAD was a primary diagnosis for all girls, although they may have had other comorbid diagnoses. There was a wait-list comparison group which was a relative strength of this study. Parents and clinicians reported improvement in the girls' symptoms post camp. In fact, after participation in camp, 50 % of the girls were not diagnosed with SAD by clinicians, whereas 100 % of girls in the wait-list group still had SAD as a primary diagnosis. Interestingly, child ratings were not consistent with those provided by parents and clinicians. Children did not report significant improvements in anxiety symptoms. The researchers concluded that this was not surprising, given that child and parent ratings can differ. However, because there was not agreement, it may be advisable to replicate or repeat the study to determine whether results would be robust in a second trial of this camp intervention.

Cobham (2012) conducted a study where children (7–14 years) were assigned to an individual treatment group, a group receiving individual treatment and bibliotherapy, and a wait-list control group. In the individual treatment group, children and parents participated in individual treatment. One therapist provided treatment sessions for each family. The intervention for children helped them to problemsolve and generate more realistic, "helpful" thoughts to cope with anxiety. Children also learned "brave" behaviors as they gradually were introduced to anxiety-provoking stimuli and overcame avoidance through graded (gradual) exposure experiences. When the child was able to experience gradual exposure to anxiety-provoking stimuli, he or she had opportunities overcome the avoidance response. The avoidance response allows the anxiety to grow or increase, so it maintains and also reinforces anxiety. In their sessions parents learned about their role in managing their child's anxiety and the anxiety management strategies that their child was learning. Many programs involve parent training. Parent training can be very effective when the parent is also experiencing anxiety (Simon et al., 2012).

Cobham (2012) also described treatment for the children and parents in the individual therapy plus bibliotherapy group. In this group there was a brief individual therapy training with a therapist, and then parents received workbooks for themselves and their child. The therapist contacted parents by telephone to discuss the workbooks and provide support (telephone contacts lasted about 12 min). Parents read their workbook, which explained their role in managing their child's anxiety and anxiety management strategies they could use with their child. Then, parents went over the program with their child, with biweekly telephone contacts with a therapist. The therapist provided support and answered questions. Results of this study indicated that both the individual therapy and individual therapy plus bibliotherapy were effective after the program had ended and at 3- and 6-month follow-up assessments. There were no appreciable differences in child functioning between the two treatment groups, and this was encouraging because the bibliotherapy group was more cost-effective and had the potential to reach more children and parents in need of treatment.

Essau et al. (2012) implemented the "FRIENDS" program, developed by Barrett and colleagues (e.g., Barrett, Farrell, Ollendick, & Dadds, 2006). The FRIENDS program is an anxiety prevention program that uses CBT interventions to assist children in coping with anxiety-provoking situations. FRIENDS is an acronym used to remind children problem-solving steps for coping with anxiety. The "F" stands for "feeling worry." The "R" is for staying relaxed. The "I" is for monitoring thinking or one's "inner thoughts" to check for negative thinking or thinking that would increase feelings of anxiety. The "E" is for exploring plans to reduce negative or anxiety-provoking thinking. The "N" is to reward or praise oneself ("nice work") for implementing plans to think positively. The "D" is for "don't forget to practice," so that children will remember to practice the coping steps outlined in FRIENDS to reduce the possibility that they might experience anxiety. Finally, the "S" is for "staying calm" and reminds children to remain calm. The program features animals to capture children's attention and it is implemented using role plays and games. There are homework exercises that allow children to practice what they learned during sessions. This has been a successful anxiety-prevention program.

Essau et al. (2012) implemented this program in 14 schools in Germany. There were intervention and control schools—as the "school" was the unit these researchers used to randomly assign children to receive the intervention or be in a wait-list control school. The wait-list control group of schools comprised children in schools who would receive the intervention after the impact of the intervention was examined for those in the intervention schools. Essau et al. believed that the FRIENDS program would result in reduced anxiety and depressive symptoms in children. The program was administered by trained graduate students who were supervised regularly. There were 302 children in the treatment group and 336 in the control group. The FRIENDS program is intensive, with about 10 weeks of treatment sessions and follow-up sessions, to boost learning, at 1 month and 3 months after the last session. Parents also learned about the program and how to help children face "feared" situations in several sessions.

Evaluation results were interesting. Essau et al. (2012) did not find differences in the children's anxious and depressive thinking immediately after the program was delivered. Yet, it was encouraging that the results of an assessment 12 months after the program ended indicated that children in the intervention group were experiencing lower levels of anxiety and depression. Encouragingly, they also discovered that children who participated in the intervention were less likely to have an "avoidant" coping style. Children who avoid feared stimuli are likely to increase their feelings of anxiety, because they are reinforcing the anxiety that they are feeling. Thus, children with a "less avoidant" coping style would be less likely to develop anxiety because they "face their fears."

CBT interventions are very successful in reducing anxiety for children. Rapee (2012) reported that approximately 50–60 % of children who participated in CBT interventions showed a reduction in anxiety symptoms immediately after participating in an intervention. Interestingly, an even greater number of children can show improvement, meaning a reduction in symptoms of anxiety, at longer intervals after treatment (up to 1 year after treatment, Rapee, 2012). On the other hand, children can experience a recurrence of symptoms, especially during times of stress. Thus, there also is relatively high chance that anxiety symptoms will recur. In fact, about half of the children who participate in CBT are likely to have a recurrence of their anxiety symptoms at some point post treatment (Hudson et al., 2014).

CBT interventions may be enhanced with computer training to decrease the "fear" or anxiety associated with neutral stimuli. Many children with anxiety ascribe fear to what others might consider to be neutral stimuli. As mentioned earlier in this chapter, Shechner et al. (2014) used an intervention where an anxiety-provoking stimulus was paired with a neutral stimulus that was not anxiety provoking through a computer task. When this type of pairing occurs, then the anxiety associated with the anxiety-provoking stimulus becomes more neutral or decreases. Over repeated trials the child's attention bias is retrained so that he or she is not always feeling anxious about a stimuli/event. Schechner et al. (2014) found that this type of intervention is a useful addition to participation in CBT. They speculated that attention bias training targets the involuntary anxiety response, while CBT targets a voluntary response to anxiety. Therefore, both types of training may be useful for treating anxiety in children.

Reynolds et al. (2012) reviewed 55 studies assessing the influence of psychotherapy for the management of anxiety disorders in children and adolescents. They reported that a majority of the studies used CBT as the therapeutic intervention. Intervening with individual children could be more effective than group treatment; but, both could have positive effects. A longer time in treatment, 11–12 sessions, can improve the impact of CBT interventions. Although treatment was effective for younger children, positive results could be even stronger for adolescents. Reynolds et al. recommended several areas for future study. For example, more research is needed to determine what type of parent involvement in child sessions is needed and to improve understanding of which components of parent treatment programs are effective. More information is needed about which CBT interventions are better for what types of anxiety disorders.

Roles for Health Educators

Health educators can play an important role in administering prevention programs in schools. Critical ideas to address in these programs are teaching children relaxation strategies and how to engage in positive self-talk. Talking positively to oneself and learning to identify and overcome negative thinking can protect children against negative thought processes, which can be synonymous with both depressive and anxious thinking styles. If children are striving for perfection, messages include "your best is good enough" and "trying your best is a special accomplishment." Health professionals need to be alert to cases in which worry interferes with child functioning and accomplishment of tasks of daily living. Children with significant levels of anxiety should be evaluated for referral to therapy. Typically, children will respond favorably to treatment, although symptoms of anxiety may recur during stressful periods. If parents are anxious or exhibit negative thought patterns and symptoms of worry, it may be beneficial to ensure that parents attend child counseling sessions or attend their own counseling in order to treat "adult anxiety." Parent behaviors may have a key role in maintaining the child's symptoms, if parents are inadvertently modeling anxious behavior. In addition to teaching children to relax and think positively, it is important to understand that graded exposure to feared events and stimuli can help a child overcome anxiety, whereas avoiding anxiety-provoking events and stimuli can actually increase anxiety by reinforcing it.

Case Study

Kara is a 7-year-old girl, who is in the second grade. She talks "constantly" at home, but not at all in her classroom. She is an only child and her parents are very, very involved in her life. They take her to all her activities and they stay "close." Her mother tends to speak for her in social situations. Kara's "not talking" at school has been a great concern and lead to a referral to see a child psychologist. Her second grade teacher, a very caring and concerned educator, has been in constant contact with her parents. Things that they (the teacher, with parent support) have used to try to get Kara to speak include praise, requesting that she talk to friends in the classroom, etc. These strategies have worked "once or twice," but lasting change has not occurred. It has not been possible to assess her reading and math skills to determine her academic abilities, which is important for moving into the third grade.

Kara attended the first therapy appointment with her parents. Initially, she remained in the waiting room with her father. Her mother provided background information. Kara was born "full term" after a normal pregnancy. She went home from the hospital the next day with her mother. Kara walked a little before 1 year of age and she was talking before the age of 2. Her mother stated that Kara met all of her developmental markers (speaking, sitting, feeding herself, walking) on time or ahead of schedule. She is a good eater and is generally very healthy. She has no major medical problems and does not take any type of medications. Her parents have noticed that she does not converse or talk to others at her gymnastics lessons or at her dance lessons. She does talk with one other little girl in her neighborhood, who she plays with regularly. In terms of helping her talk at school, her parents have tried to encourage her, scold her, and lately taken away privileges when she continued to refuse to try to talk at school. They also have had many "heart-to-heart talks" with Kara to encourage talking. They were becoming fearful that the talks would damage their relationship with their daughter.

After background information was obtained, the child psychologist met with Kara and her parents. Kara's mother tended to talk for her and her daughter clung to her side. Her mother described that Kara could be shy when meeting others and rarely talked to other adults. Kara talked with her mother using gestures and by nodding her head. For example, she would shake her head up and down to indicate "yes," if her mother correctly interpreted her feelings. Her mother was very practiced at reading Kara's facial expressions and knowing what she might be going to say. Therefore, it was relatively easy for Kara's mother to "talk for her" during the session. Kara's father was quiet and admitted that he had experienced anxiety as a youth and was very shy as a youngster. In fact, he stated that, "I'm still shy today and I can become very nervous about how others are evaluating my work."

After observing and interacting with Kara and her parents, the child psychologist asked to speak again with Kara's parents. Kara played in a nearby waiting room. The child psychologist mentioned that Kara's mother appeared to be talking for her, so much so that Kara did not need to talk to express her needs. Kara's mother was defensive at first, mentioning that she needed to help her daughter communicate to others. After a bit more conversation had occurred, her mother did admit that she was talking for Kara. The child psychologist discussed how her mother could ignore the tugs on her arm sleeve and looks from Kara, so that Kara would have to talk more for herself. Kara's father, who was quietly listening to the conversation, offered to help Kara's mother by reminding her not to talk for Kara.

As the conversation progressed, Kara's father talked about the fact that he would like to be involved in helping Kara learn to "speak up" for herself in social situations. He agreed to role play—three times weekly—Kara talking with her teacher and peers at school. The child psychologist also developed a reward chart, where Kara would receive a prize—time to play games with her mother and father—should she talk with her teacher in the classroom or say "hi" to another student. Kara's parents agreed to provide this behavior chart to Kara's teacher. They would ask the teacher to send a note home from school daily, so that Kara's parents could provide her with a reward and lots of praise if she spoke with others at school. In addition, Kara's father signed a "Release of Information Form" that would allow the child psychologist to discuss Kara's school performance and share information with Kara's teacher.

When the child psychologist called Kara's teacher, they talked about her performance at school. Her teacher reported that she could not be sure of Kara's academic level, because she could not complete her testing. Upon further questioning, her teacher did state that Kara's homework was done correctly and that her class assignments were completed, even though Kara was often late or needed extra time to complete class assignments. The child psychologist discussed Kara's academic potential with the teacher and they both agreed that she was probably on target for moving to the next grade level. Both thought that Kara was of average intelligence. The child psychologist agreed to write a brief letter to the school team in charge of promoting the children to the next grade, outlining her impressions of Kara's intellectual functioning and academic skills based on teacher and parent report. The teacher hoped that this report might provide evidence that Kara was showing "readiness" to move to the next grade level, even though she did not complete the standardized tests with her teacher.

Further counseling sessions with Kara were positive. She was able to speak with her child psychologist. Kara responded positively to the reward chart. In time, Kara was able to speak to her teacher in the classroom, typically responding to a question from her teacher. She was able to say "hello" to her classmates and say "Can I play with you?" on the playground. Her teacher and Kara's father did not feel thrilled with Kara's progress. The child psychologist worked to educate them about the slow progress (slow gains in improving talking and interacting with others) of children who were not talkative in social settings. She pointed to the difference in Kara's emotions—Kara was more upbeat and happy when coming home, because she was talking when her teacher initiated a conversation with her. The therapist reviewed the progress over the course of a month, from no talking to daily talking. After this review, Kara's father and teacher became more "relaxed" about Kara's progress. This was positive for Kara, because she flourished as the adults around her became more relaxed about her progress. Kara's teacher and her father agreed that the reward chart was working and that although gains were slow, they were seeing improvement in Kara's "responding to others" in school. She was smiling more in school, which also made her peers more likely to invite her to play with them and join them in completing classroom activities.

Kara's mother was thrilled with her daughter's progress. She had been very shy as a child, and although she was able to talk to others more easily as an adult, her mother empathized with Kara a great deal. The therapist and her mother discussed her empathy for her daughter and how this empathy might influence Kara's mother to talk for her in different situations. They discussed that her mother should try to ignore Kara's tugs on her sleeve and eye gestures that meant that she wanted her mother to answer for her. After some discussion, Kara's mother admitted that she might be enabling Kara's lack of conversation by talking for her in different social situations. She agreed to look away and ask Kara to talk for herself. At first this plan was not successful and was very stressful for Kara's mother. After a few weeks, her mother became more "practiced" at not responding to Kara's bids for her mother to talk for her. Kara, although initially upset with her mother, became more acclimated to her mother's silent insistence that she speak for herself. After a period of a few weeks, Kara did talk for herself a few times when her mother was ignoring her signals to talk for her. Kara was very pleased with herself when she did initiate a conversation with another child at a playground in their neighborhood.

Over time, Kara was able to order from the children's menu in a restaurant. She was able to speak with her coach in her gymnastics lessons. She was able to say "hello" to other young girls who also attended her gymnastics class. She even talked more with her grandmother. This was a source for celebration in the family, because her grandmother had been very upset that Kara was not speaking with her.

After 6 months of bi-weekly therapy sessions, Kara's mother and father believed that Kara's progress was advanced to a level that she could take a "summer break" from therapy sessions. Kara was excited for this break. She said a break would be beneficial, since she worried that something was wrong with her because she had to attend therapy. The therapist had assured her that she was very smart and had many positive traits. Unfortunately, Kara still worried that she was not "normal" because she had to see a therapist. The therapist was used to this "stigma" or negative attitude about coming to therapy sessions. The therapist handled Kara's reaction well, pointing out Kara's strengths and the fact that many children and adults have "trouble spots" they need to work on in therapy. She pointed out all of Kara's gains, in terms of talking to others and interacting with them, as evidence of her progress in therapy. Kara seemed to brighten with this information. Both of Kara's parents agreed to "check in" with or contact the therapist at the end of the summer to determine if further therapy would be needed when the school year resumed in August. They were pleased with Kara's progress and worked with the therapist to develop a reward chart for tracking her socialization at her summer camp. Her mother agreed that she would continue her plan to "not talk for my daughter."

Summary

In this chapter, definitions for different types of child anxiety were reviewed. Treatment of this problem can be successful, although children may re-experience anxiety at a later point in time. Interventions involve changing negative thinking, which can be beliefs that things will not turn out well or putting pressure on oneself to "get the job perfect." Relaxation and breathing can help the child cope with physiological arousal that often occurs when he or she is feeling anxious. Graded exposure, where children gradually learn to move through anxious thinking and confront and master anxious situations can be helpful in reducing the anxiety children feel. Avoiding situations, events, or stimuli that make the child feel anxious can actually increase feelings of anxiety, by reinforcing them. Involving parents in treatment can be helpful, especially if parents are anxious. Health educators should refer children with high anxiety levels for treatment by a child psychologist or other experienced mental health professionals. Prevention programs in schools may hold promise for teaching children how to reduce "anxiety-prone" thinking, such as thinking things are their fault and they have to be perfect. Learning about the impact of internet-based interventions to reduce child anxiety and reach parents may be important, as many children are in need of treatment and may not be able to access clinic-based care.

Exercises/Review Questions
1. Define obsessive-compulsive disorder.
2. What are your ideas for using graded exposure (exposing a child in a step-by-step, slow fashion) to help a child deal with his or her fears of socializing with peers during an after-school activity?

   (a) Share your ideas for helping the child practice (i.e., graded exposure) and your ideas for charting or keeping track of progress.
   (b) Would you reward the child for practicing or for actually talking with others?
   (c) What types of rewards might you use?

3. If you were asked to design a training session to educate teachers about helping children with anxiety, what would be key components of your session? What key educational topics would you address and why?
4. Let's think about the FRIENDS acronym. Do you believe the steps in the FRIENDS acronym address key factors that would help a child reduce feelings of anxiety?
5. What was the diagnosis for Kara (presented in the case study)? What symptoms did you notice that informed your diagnostic impression?
6. Do you believe Kara's parents were experiencing anxiety? If yes, do you have any ideas for treating her parents?

Key Concepts
Separation Anxiety Disorder
Generalized Anxiety Disorder
Social Anxiety Disorder
Obsessive Compulsive Disorder
Challenging anxious thinking
Positive self-talk
Avoidance cycle
External locus of control
State of hyperarousal
Exposure to feared stimuli
Coping Cat Program
BRAVE intervention
FRIENDS intervention

References

Abramowitz, J. S., Taylor, S., & McKay, D. (2009). Obsessive-compulsive disorder. *Lancet, 374*(9688), 491–499.

Albano, A. M., & Kendall, P. C. (2002). Cognitive behavioural therapy for children and adolescents with anxiety disorders: Clinical research advances. *International Review of Psychiatry, 14*(2), 129–134. doi:10.1080/09540260220132644.

Allen, J. L., Rapee, R. M., & Sanberg, S. (2008). Severe life events and chronic adversities as antecedents to anxiety in children: A matched control study. *Journal of Abnormal Child Psychology, 36*, 1047–1056.

American Psychiatric Association. (2013). *Diagnostic and statistical manual of mental disorders* (5th ed.). Washington, DC: Author.

Barlow, D. H. (2002). *Anxiety and its disorders: The nature and treatment of anxiety and panic* (2nd ed.). New York, NY: Guilford.

Barrett, P. M., Farrell, L. J., Ollendick, T. H., & Dadds, M. (2006). Long-term outcomes of an Australian universal prevention trial of anxiety and depression symptoms in children and youth: An evaluation of the friends program. *Journal of Clinical Child and Adolescent Psychology, 35*(3), 403–411.

Biederman, J., Hirshfeld-Becker, D. R., Rosenbaum, J. F., Hérot, C., Friedman, D., Snidman, N., … Faraone, S. V. (2001). Further evidence of association between behavioral inhibition and social anxiety in children. *American Journal of Psychiatry, 158*(10), 1673–1679. Retrieved June 13, 2015, from http://dx.doi.org/10.1176/appi.ajp.158.10.1673.

Clark, L. A., & Watson, D. (1991). Tripartite model of anxiety and depression: Psychometric evidence and taxonomic implications. *Journal of Abnormal Psychology, 107*, 74–85.

Cobham, V. E. (2012). Do anxiety-disordered children need to come into clinic for efficacious treatment? *Journal of Consulting and Clinical Psychology, 80*(3), 465–476.

Copeland, W. E., Angold, A., Shanahan, L., & Costello, E. (2014). Longitudinal patterns of anxiety from childhood to adulthood: The Great Smokey Mountains Study. *Journal of the American Academy of Child and Adolescent Psychiatry, 53*(1), 21–33.

Costello, E. J., Egger, H. L., & Angold, A. (2005). The developmental epidemiology of anxiety disorders: Phenomenology, prevalence, and comorbidity. *Child and Adolescent Psychiatric Clinics of North America, 14*(4), 631–648.

Creswell, C., Waite, P., & Cooper, P. J. (2014). Assessment and management of anxiety disorders in children and adolescents. *Archives of Disease in Childhood, 99*, 674–678. doi:10.1136/archdischild-2013-303768.

Degnan, K. A., Almas, A. N., & Fox, N. A. (2010). Temperament and the environment in the etiology of childhood anxiety. *Journal of Child Psychology and Psychiatry, 51*(4), 497–517.

Drake, K. L., & Ginsburg, G. S. (2012). Family factors and the development, treatment, and prevention of childhood anxiety disorders. *Clinical Child and Family Psychology Review, 15*, 144–162. doi:10.1007/s10567-011-0109-0.

Essau, C. A., Conradt, J., Sasagawa, S., & Ollendick, T. H. (2012). Prevention of anxiety symptoms in children: Results from a universal school-based trial. *Behavior Therapy, 43*, 450–464.

Fonseca, A. C., & Perrin, S. (2011). The clinical phenomenology and classification of child and adolescent anxiety. In W. K. Silverman & A. P. Field (Eds.), *Anxiety disorders in children and adolescents* (2nd ed., pp. 25–55). Cambridge, UK: Cambridge University Press.

Grover, R. L., Ginsburg, G. S., & Ialongo, N. (2007). Childhood predictors of anxiety: A longitudinal study. *Child Psychiatry and Human Development, 36*(2), 133–153.

Herbert, M. (2013). Etiological considerations. In T. H. Ollendick, N. J. King, & W. Yule (Eds.), *International handbook of phobic and anxiety disorders in children and adolescents* (pp. 3–20). New York, NY: Springer.

Holly, L. E., Little, M., Pina, A. A., & Caterino, L. C. (2015). Assessment of anxiety symptoms in school children: A cross sex and ethnic examination. *Journal of Abnormal Child Psychology, 43*(2), 297–309.

Hudson, J. L., Newall, C., Rapee, R. M., Lyneham, H. J., Schniering, C. C., Wuthrich, V. M., …
Gar, N. S. (2014). The impact of brief parental anxiety management on child anxiety treatment
outcomes: A controlled trial. *Journal of Clinical Child and Adolescent Psychology, 43*(3),
370–380. doi: 10.1080/15374416.2013.807734.

Kahn, J., Nursten, J. P., & Carroll, H. C. M. (1981). *Unwillingly to school: School phobia or school
refusal: A psychosocial problem* (3rd ed.). Elmsford, NY: Pergamon Press.

Kendall, P. C. (1994). Treating anxiety disorders in children: Results of a randomized clinical trial.
Journal of Consulting and Clinical Psychology, 62, 100–110.

Kendall, P. C. (2012). Anxiety disorders in youth. In P. Kendall (Ed.), *Child and adolescent therapy: Cognitive-behavioral procedures* (4th ed., pp. 143–189). New York, NY: The Guilford
Press.

Kendall, P. C., Flannery-Schroeder, E., Panichelli-Mindel, S., Southam-Gerow, M., Henin, A., &
Warman, M. (1997). Therapy for youths with anxiety disorders: A second randomized clinical
trial. *Journal of Consulting and Clinical Psychology, 65*(3), 366–380.

Kendall, P. C., & Hedtke, K. A. (2006a). *Cognitive-behavioral therapy for anxious children:
Therapist manual* (3rd ed.). Ardmore, PA: Workbook Publishing.

Kendall, P. C., & Hedtke, K. A. (2006b). *The coping cat workbook* (2nd ed.). Ardmore, PA:
Workbook Publishing.

March, S., Spence, S. H., & Donovan, C. L. (2009). The efficacy of an internet-based cognitive-
behavioral therapy intervention for child anxiety disorders. *Journal of Pediatric Psychology,
34*(5), 474–487.

Maynard, B. R., Brendel, K., Bulanda, J. J., Heyne, D., Thompson, A., & Pigott, T. (2015).
Psychosocial interventions for school refusal with primary and secondary school students: A
systematic review. *Campbell Systematic Reviews, 11*(12).

Merikangas, K. R., He, M. J. P., Burstein, M., Swanson, M. S. A., Avenevoli, S., Cui, M. L., …
Swendsen, J. (2010). Lifetime prevalence of mental disorders in US adolescents: Results from
the National Comorbidity Study-Adolescent Supplement (NCS-A). *Journal of the American
Academy of Child and Adolescent Psychiatry, 49*(10), 980–989. doi: 10.1016/j.jaac.2010.05.017.

Norman, K. R., Silverman, W. K., & Lebowitz, E. R. (2015). Family accommodation of child and
adolescent anxiety: Mechanisms, assessment, and treatment. *Journal of Child and Adolescent
Psychiatric Nursing, 28*(3), 131–140.

Ollendick, T. H., Costa, N. M., & Benoit, K. E. (2010). Interpersonal processes and the anxiety
disorders of childhood. In G. Beck (Ed.), *Interpersonal processes in the anxiety disorders:
Implications for understanding psychopathology and treatment* (pp. 71–95). Washington, DC:
American Psychological Association.

Ollendick, T. H., Halldorsdottir, T., Fraire, M. G., Austin, K. E., Noguchi, R. J., Lewis, K. M., …
Whitmore, M. J. (2015). Specific phobias in youth: A randomized controlled trial comparing
one-session treatment to a parent-augmented one-session treatment. *Behavior Therapy, 46*(2),
141–155. doi: 10.1016/j.beth.2014.09.004.

Rapee, R. M. (2012). F. 1. Anxiety disorders in children and adolescents: Nature, development,
treatment, and prevention. In J. M. Rey (Ed.), *Section F. Anxiety disorders of the IACAPAP
e-textbook of child and adolescent mental health* (pp. 1–19). Geneva, Switzerland: International
Association for Child and Adolescent Psychiatry and Allied Professions.

Reynolds, S., Wilson, C., Austin, J., & Hooper, L. (2012). Effects of psychotherapy for anxiety in
children and adolescents: A meta-analytic review. *Clinical Psychology Review, 32*, 251–262.

Santucci, L. C., & Ehrenreich-May, J. (2013). A randomized controlled trial of the child anxiety
multi-day program (CAMP) for separation anxiety disorder. *Child Psychiatry & Human
Development, 44*(3), 439–451. doi:10.1007/s10578-012-0338-6.

Shechner, T., Rimon-Chakis, A., Britton, J. C., Lotan, D., Apter, A., Bliese, P. D., … Bar-Haim, Y.
(2014). Attention bias modification treatment augmenting effects on cognitive-behavioral therapy in children with anxiety: Randomized controlled trial. *Journal of the American Academy
of Child and Adolescent Psychiatry, 53*(1), 61–71.

Silverman, W. K., & Albano, A. M. (1996). *The anxiety disorders interview schedule for DSM-IV—
Child and parent versions.* San Antonio, TX: Psychological Corporation.

Simon, E., Dirksen, C., Bögels, S., & Bodden, D. (2012). Cost-effectiveness of child-focused and parent-focused interventions in a child anxiety prevention program. *Journal of Anxiety Disorders, 26*, 287–296.

Spence, S. H. (1997). Structure of anxiety symptoms among children: A confirmatory factor-analytic study. *Journal of Abnormal Psychology, 106*(2), 280–297.

Spence, S. H. (1998). A measure of anxiety symptoms among children. *Behaviour Research and Therapy, 36*(5), 545–566.

Spence, S. H., Holmes, J. M., March, S., & Lipp, O. V. (2006). The feasibility and outcome of clinic plus internet delivery of cognitive behavior therapy for childhood anxiety. *Journal of Consulting and Clinical Psychology, 74*(3), 614–621.

Torp, N. C., Dahl, K., Skarphedinsson, G., Thomsen, P. H., Valderhaug, R., Weidle, B., … Ivarsson, T. (2015). Effectiveness of cognitive behavior treatment for pediatric Obsessive-Compulsive Disorder: Acute outcomes from the Nordic long-term OCD treatment study (NordLOTS). *Behaviour Research and Therapy, 64*, 15–23.

Vasey, M. W., Bosmans, G., & Ollendick, T. H. (2014). The developmental psychopathology of anxiety. In M. Lewis & K. D. Rudolph (Eds.), *Handbook of developmental psychopathology* (3rd ed., pp. 543–560). New York, NY: Springer.

Chapter 8
Depression

Ashley Merianos

Diagnosis

In the *Diagnostic and Statistical Manual of Mental Disorders, Fifth Edition* (DSM-5), depressive disorders have in common the experience of a sad emotional state or sad affect (American Psychiatric Association, 2013). Children may also display irritable moods when they feel depressed. Further, children who are experiencing depression may exhibit cognitive (such as difficulty concentrating) and physical symptoms (such as lethargy) that make it difficult for them to function as they normally would. In the DSM-5, depressive disorders are separated from bipolar and other related disorders which may involve other states, such as mania, or periods of elation when one may have difficulty sleeping. This chapter will focus on three diagnostic categories: Major Depressive Disorder, Disruptive Mood Dysregulation Disorder, and Persistent Depressive Disorder.

Major Depressive Disorder. Similar to adults, children can experience major depressive disorder. This involves significant feelings of depressed mood and loss of interest or pleasure in usual activities. The child may feel hopeless and sad and may display irritable mood. There is a loss of interest and experience of pleasure in most daily activities. The depressed mood and loss of interest in pleasurable activities occurs daily for a 2-week period and should represent a change from the child's previous level of functioning. In addition to the aforementioned major symptoms, major depressive disorder can also be accompanied by significant weight change (either loss or gain), change in sleeping behaviors (e.g., insomnia, hypersomnia), fatigue, change in psychomotor functioning (either retardation or agitation), and diminished abilities to think clearly and concentrate. A child who is experiencing major depression may feel that he or she wants to die and feel worthless. Making decisions and completing

---

The original version of this chapter was revised. An erratum to this chapter can be found at DOI 10.1007/978-3-319-31117-3_12

L. Nabors, *Medical and Mental Health During Childhood*, Springer
Series on Child and Family Studies, DOI 10.1007/978-3-319-31117-3_8

school work may be very difficult. Major depressive disorder may appear at any age, but becomes more likely after children experience puberty. When making this diagnosis, the clinician also specifies whether the child is experiencing mild, moderate, or severe depression and whether there are multiple or recurrent episodes versus a single episode of depression (American Psychiatric Association, 2013).

Disruptive Mood Dysregulation Disorder. The DSM-5 added a new diagnosis entitled, "Disruptive Mood Dysregulation Disorder," for children with irritable mood who also have difficulty controlling their emotions and behaviors. Children with this disorder are likely to develop unipolar depression or anxiety disorder as they become adolescents (American Psychiatric Association, 2013). Dougherty et al. (2014) stated that this diagnosis is characterized by severe and chronic irritable mood and temper tantrums that are significant and inconsistent with the situations in which the child finds him- or herself. The temper tantrums are not what might be expected for the child's age or developmental level and must occur at least three times a week. The child's mood is consistently irritable and angry for 12 months in at least two settings (most notably in home and school contexts). This disorder cannot be diagnosed before 6 years of age and must be diagnosed before 10 years of age. Dougherty et al. (2014) also mentioned that this new diagnosis has caused some controversy, in terms of whether it should be a diagnosis. The reason is that it shares symptoms with many disorders, such as Oppositional Defiant Disorder, Attention Deficit-Hyperactivity Disorder, and Bipolar Disorder. Because this diagnosis is somewhat controversial, and has relatively less emphasis in scientific literature, information on this disorder will not be featured as prominently in this chapter.

Persistent Depressive Disorder. Children who have experienced symptoms of depression for a year also may be diagnosed with Persistent Depressive Disorder or Dysthymic Disorder (Dysthymia). Children with this diagnosis experience long-standing feelings of sadness—for 1 year or longer. The child will have experienced depressed mood more days than not for a year (American Psychiatric Association, 2013). In adults, the symptoms will need to have occurred for 2 years. The child will have experienced similar symptoms to those listed for major depressive disorder including low self-esteem, feelings of hopelessness, changes in appetite and sleep patterns, fatigue, and difficulty concentrating and making decisions. Children with Persistent Depressive Disorder may also experience a major depressive episode during the same period in which they experience long-standing sadness. In addition, a major depressive episode may precede the development of dysthymic disorder or persistent depressive disorder. Similar to Major Depressive Disorder, children with Persistent Depressive Disorder may experience other mental health problems, such as anxiety and substance abuse problems.

Prevalence of Depression in Children

Up to 2.8 % children in the United States are estimated to have a depressive disorder (Birmaher et al., 1996; Costello, Erkanli, & Angold, 2006). Studies of prevalence for child depression have used multiple assessments, contributing to different estimates of prevalence of depression in this population (Kessler, Avenevoli, & Ries Merikangas, 2001). Further, depression in preschool aged children from 3 to 6 years shows prevalence rates of between 1 and 2 %, which is similar to rates for school aged children (Egger & Angold, 2006; Luby, Heffelfinger, & Mrakotsky, 2003). Trends show that the prevalence of depression increases with age.

Although children may not meet the diagnostic criteria for a depressive disorder, they may have subclinical levels of symptoms. For example, a study among 11–16-year-old females revealed that 6 % had a major depressive disorder in the past year and more than one-fifth (20.7 %) of 11–16-year-olds exhibited partial symptomatology, but did not meet the DSM criteria for a depressive disorder (Cooper & Goodyer, 1993). The developmental course of this disease is bimodal in nature with an increase at 11 years of age and again increasing after 15 years of age, leveling out from 18 to 26 years of age (Kim-Cohen et al., 2003). Research indicates the probability for recurrence of depression is anywhere from 20 to 60 % 1–2 years after remission and peaks to 70 % after 5 years of remission from a major depressive episode over time (Birmaher et al., 1996; Costello et al., 2002). Remission is a temporary end to symptoms. The prevalence of this disease is lower among children compared to adolescents, with up to 25 % lifetime prevalence in late adolescence; evidence shows that the onset of major depressive disorders typically occur between mid to late adolescence and early adulthood (Kessler et al., 2001).

Gender differences typically do not exist among children, but occur later in life during adolescence and young adulthood. Multiple studies have found that the male/female ratio of diagnosed depression in children is about equal, but in male and female adolescents and adults is 1:2 (Birmaher et al., 1996; Kessler, McGonagle, Swartz, Blazer, & Nelson, 1993). This sex ratio does not emerge until sometime between 10 and 15 years of age, and the risk for depression increases significantly after puberty, especially in females (Angold & Costello, 2006).

Racial/ethnic group differences of depression diagnoses remain unclear in children. However, national research indicates that adults reporting two or more races (11.4 %) had highest rates of a past year major depressive episode followed by 8.9 % American Indians or Alaska Natives, 7.3 % whites, 5.8 % Hispanics, 4.6 % African Americans, 4.0 % Asians, and 1.6 % Native Hawaiian or Other Pacific Islanders (Substance Abuse and Mental Health Services Administration, 2014). Another US epidemiologic study found that white adults (11.2 %) were more likely to have reported any depressive disorder in the past 12 months compared to their Hispanic (10.8 %), African-American (8.0 %), and Asian (5.4 %) adult counterparts (Alegría et al., 2008). Similar to adults, rates of past year major depressive episodes in adolescents were reported in 8.7 % of whites, 8.4 % of Hispanics, 7.4 % of Asians, and 7.3 % of African-Americans (Cummings & Druss, 2011).

The relationship between low socioeconomic status (SES) and depression has been well documented in adult populations (Lorant et al., 2003), but this relationship is inconclusive in children. Several studies have found that SES is associated with depression in children (Goodman, Huang, Wade, & Kahn, 2003; Kubik, Lytle, Birnbaum, Murray, & Perry, 2003; Tracy, Zimmerman, Galea, McCauley, & Stoep,

2008). Contrarily, research found no relationship between SES and depressive symptoms in 10-year-olds (Leech, Larkby, Day, & Day, 2006).

Genetic and Environmental Determinants. Genetic and environmental factors are attributed in the etiology (cause) of depression. Studies have found that diagnosable depression, including major depressive disorders, is a familial disorder, which is influenced by the interaction of genetic and environmental determinants (Caspi et al., 2003; Kendler, Kuhn, Vittum, Prescott, & Riley, 2005; Pilowsky, Wickramaratne, Nomura, & Weissman, 2006; Weissman et al., 2005). Weissman et al. (2005) conducted a longitudinal retrospective cohort, family study to examine the relationship between familial mental disorders and functioning in three generations and found that diagnosis rates are highest in grandchildren of parents and grandparents with a moderate to severe major depressive disorder impairment. A longitudinal study means that participants are studied over time and data are collected at multiple points in time (e.g., participants completing a survey once every year for 5 years in a row). A cohort study is defined as a group of people who share a characteristic at a specific time (e.g., date of depressive disorder diagnosis). Thus, family loading has been underscored as the primary predictive factor associated with the risk of developing a major depressive disorder (Nomura, Wickramaratne, Warner, Mufson, & Weissman, 2002; Weissman et al., 2005).

Environmental determinants that influence childhood depression have also been documented. For example, Pilowsky et al. (2006) assessed the effects parental depression and family discord had on psychopathology among children at high and low risk of depression and found that parental depression is related to family discord and is a prominent factor related to major depressive disorders in children. A longitudinal study that followed children at risk for depression over time tested the relationship between acute and chronic stress and depression and found that chronic family stress at 15 years old predicted higher depression scores at 20 years old (Hammen, Brennan, Keenan-Miller, Hazel, & Najman, 2010).

The onset of depression may be moderated or mediated by several influences. It is important to note that a review of the literature found there are sizeable age differences in neurobiological correlates existing between children, adolescents, and adults (Kaufman, Martin, King, & Charney, 2001). Pine, Cohen, Johnson, and Brook (2002) found that adverse child life events (e.g., school failure, physical abuse in the home) predicted an increased risk for depression in early adulthood. Other stressors that contribute to the development and maintenance of depressive symptoms in children include, but are not limited to, biological factors, sociocultural factors, life events (e.g., changes in school status, changes in physical health), and comorbid disorders (e.g., substance abuse, ADHD, and anxiety disorders) (Caspi et al., 2003; Costello et al., 2002; Kaufman et al., 2001; Kendler et al., 2005; Pine et al., 2002; Weissman et al., 2005). It should be noted that the impact these stressors have on a child depends on the child's way of thinking about what is happening to him or her. If the child has a negative attributional style or a catastrophizing style, always thinking that the worst will occur, then this can make it more difficult for him or her to cope with stress that can lead to depressed thoughts. This negative attribution style has been associated with depression (Angold, Costello, & Erkanli, 1999).

Impact for Children

This chapter focuses on how depression impacts children based on Bronfenbrenner's Ecological Systems Theory. This means that a focus is to show that the child, parent(s), and family, as well as the school system are key players for implementing interventions to help the child. To this end, information will be offered to assist health professionals who work with children who experience major depressive disorder, disruptive mood dysregulation disorder, and persistent mood disorder. The overarching goal is to assist health educators and health specialists in identifying, referring, and providing coping strategies to children who are diagnosed with depression, regardless of their specific type of disorder. Although several issues remain regarding how to achieve the best health outcomes for children with a depressive disorder, this chapter will focus on treatments specifically designed for depressive disorders that are based on empirical evidence and clinical consensus.

Depressive disorders often co-occur with other psychiatric conditions. The most common comorbid diagnoses are anxiety disorders, disruptive disorders, attention-deficit/hyperactivity disorder (ADHD), and substance use disorders (Angold et al., 1999; Birmaher et al., 1996; Fombonne, Wostear, Cooper, Harrington, & Rutter, 2001; Lewinsohn, Rohde, & Seeley, 1998). Depression and anxiety are the most common comorbid or co-occurring conditions and they can both result in negative mood and feelings and negative thinking for children (Angold et al., 1999). Typically, child anxiety disorders precede depressive disorders (Avenevoli, Stolar, Li, Dierker, & Ries Merikangas, 2001). Approximately, 25–50 % of children with a depressive disorder also have an anxiety disorder and approximately 10–15 % of children with an anxiety disorder have a depressive disorder (Axelson & Birmaher, 2001).

Children with depressive disorders are at increased risk for negative life events, physical complaints (such as headaches and stomach aches), substance abuse, legal issues, and poor academic, family, and psychosocial functioning (Fergusson & Woodward, 2002; Hammen, Shih, Altman, & Brennan, 2003; Lewinsohn, Rohde, Seeley, Klein, & Gotlib, 2003). Psychosocial difficulties may persist after the remission of a depressive episode, highlighting the need for treating depression and psychosocial issues simultaneously (Fergusson & Woodward, 2002; Lewinsohn et al., 2003). Depressive disorders are likely to recur throughout an individual's life course; consequently, a disproportionate amount of children's depressive disorders will continue into adulthood. For example, children with persistent depressive disorder or dysthymia typically face a prolonged course of an estimated three to 4 years in community and clinical samples, and are at risk for future major depressive disorders (Kovacs, Akiskal, Gatsonis, & Parrone, 1994; Lewinsohn, Rohde, Seeley, & Hops, 1991).

Assessment of Depression

Currently, there are no laboratory tests to diagnose depression in children. A comprehensive psychiatric diagnostic assessment should be used to diagnose depressive disorders. Clinical assessment typically occurs in three steps: (1) diagnosis and prognosis, (2) planning of treatment, and (3) monitoring and evaluation of treatment (Klein, Dougherty, & Olino, 2005). While conducting an assessment of depression, the clinician and/or researcher must assess key symptoms. Klein et al. (2005) indicate it is important to assess any preceding course of depression, comorbid psychiatric and medical conditions, and any areas of psychosocial impairment to determine the diagnosis. Data collected during the interview are critical for treatment planning including making decisions on treatment setting and intensity and duration of treatment. The final phase of assessment entails monitoring and evaluating whether treatment should be continued or changed based on the change in symptoms and child functioning.

The two major methods for assessing depression in children are interviews and rating scales. Direct interviews should include children and their parents and potentially other informants such as teachers, primary care providers, and peers. Structured interviews can be used to assess childhood depression, but are more comprehensive in nature compared to unstructured interviews (Klein et al., 2005). A commonly used structured interview is the Child and Adolescent Psychiatric Assessment (CAPA). This structured interview includes questions about onset dates (i.e., when depressed feelings began), duration, frequency and intensity of depression, and other psychiatric diagnoses according to the *DSM* criteria (Angold & Costello, 2000). There is a child and parent-self report version of CAPA.

The most common survey for rating childhood depression is the Children's Depression Rating Scale which contains 17 items on cognitive, somatic, affective (i.e., emotions), and psychomotor symptoms (Poznanski & Mokros, 1999). This scale takes approximately 15–20 min to complete. It is important to note that a survey or scale should not be the sole instrument for diagnosing depression; detailed interviews and information from parents, children, and in some cases teachers should be obtained. This scale is available several places, including from Western Psychological Services (http://www.wpspublish.com/store/p/2703/childrens-depression-rating-scale-revised-cdrs-r, accessed January 1, 2016).

When making a decision about whether a child might be experiencing depressive symptoms, there are several questions that are important to review. The first is to determine when symptoms began (i.e., symptom onset). Health educators should ask parents and the child, if possible, to estimate symptom severity, and whether symptoms occur every day. It may be beneficial to ask the child and parent how many days a week that the child feels sad. Questions to assess whether there are changes in eating and sleeping patterns are important, as changes in both areas can occur. If the child is more withdrawn and disengaging from social activities, these can be other changes in behavior that accompany depression and dysthymic disorder. When a child is experiencing sadness, it is crucial to ask whether the child has expressed wishes to die or to kill him- or herself. If the child has expressed a wish to kill him- or herself, then the clinician needs to ask the child if he or she has any type of plan for self-harm. Assessment of previous attempts to self-harm or commit suicide should be examined. If the child indicates significant suicidal ideation (thinking about committing suicide), significant feelings of sadness consistent with dysthymic disorder or major depressive disorder, or has tried to kill him- or herself, it is recommended that referral to a licensed mental health counselor be made, so that a thorough assessment of depressive symptomatology can be conducted. It can be difficult to determine if referral is needed, but if in doubt, it is better to refer for a more thorough evaluation of the child's symptoms and previous behaviors. If there is any indication that the child is very depressed or may self-harm, evaluation in an emergency room may be warranted.

Disease Management

Disease management typically involves referral for counseling for young children. After assessment of symptoms and referral, the child and his or her parents typically begin a course of treatment with a licensed mental health counselor. Medications can also be used to treat children and more information about medication management is outlined in the next section of this chapter. Children can typically participate in either group or individual therapy or counseling. It is recommended that parents spend time with the counselor, learning how to address sadness and to identify serious behaviors that would indicate any need for immediate emergency treatment either at an emergency room or a psychiatric facility. While participating in counseling, the child may work with a therapist to cope with grief, sadness, or to recover from negative life experiences, such as trauma. The counselor will work with the child to help him or her improve negative views of the self, world, and future. Children who are experiencing depression typically see themselves in a very negative light, and they may have a negative outlook about their family and school experiences. They may not see much hope for the future.

   Children and parents need to understand their depression and symptoms related to their sadness, and education is another important goal for counseling. Depressive symptoms typically are classified into two categories: psychological and physical/somatic. The *International Classification of Mental and Behavioral Disorders System* (ICD-10) reported the top three depressive symptoms as being: (1) sad mood, (2) anhedonia or loss of pleasure in activities, and (3) decreased energy leading to fatigue (World Health Organization, 2015). It is critical for children to understand common psychological symptoms of depression, including but not limited to, sad mood, and loss of pleasure in daily activities, decreased concentration, and self-esteem, feelings of guilt or worthlessness, and suicidal ideation (thinking about dying or being dead). Children should also be taught the physical symptoms including altered sleep patterns including insomnia (i.e., reduced sleep) or hypersomnia (i.e., increased sleep), changes in appetite and/or weight, fatigue, and psycho-motor activity changes that manifest as agitation, hyperactivity, and/or anxiety. Understanding symptoms will help children identify triggers for their depressive episodes. When children understand their symptoms, they can know when to ask for help.

The therapist may often use cognitive-behavioral techniques to help the child relieve symptoms of depression. These types of treatments have a significant evidence base (i.e., support in the scientific literature) and are featured in this chapter. However, the author notes that other treatments may also be effective in helping children relieve symptoms of depression. Cognitive techniques include helping a child to challenge negative thinking or unrealistic ways of thinking. For example, if a child is feeling that he or she is not good at anything, the therapist might work with the child and parent to make a list of positive things about the child and list his or her skills to help the child to reconsider his or her value. If a child is likely to be too hard on him- or herself, the therapist may help the child to change self-talk to more positive statements. Thus, rather than saying "I should have done this," the child could say, "I tried my best and I did this well and I can improve on ____ in the future." Changing negative self-statements or negative self-talk, into positive statements and self-talk, is a key goal for improving negative thought patterns. Another technique a child can implement is positive imagery. A child can think of a "happy place" to go to when he or she is feeling sad. The child can also engage in new hobbies that are more rewarding and fun. The child needs to learn that he or she needs to be an active "agent" in working to defeat negative thinking and involve him- or herself in activities that are fun and rewarding (Field, Seligman, & Albrecht, 2008; McLaughlin & Christner, 2012).

Children who experience depression may be very reactive to stressful events in their lives. In order to help children cope better with stress, they can learn stress reduction activities, such as counting to ten before they talk about their feelings, taking ten deep breaths in a row to relax, or they can learn to use a journal as a stress management tool. Journaling provides an outlet for expressing difficult emotions (e.g., anger) and negative thoughts and has the potential to help children identify what they are feeling. Another technique to manage depression is to stop negative thinking to reduce ruminating (i.e., replay things over in the mind repeatedly). A child with a depressive disorder can be taught positive self-talk as described above.

Parents are also taught to help children be more positive (e.g., to use positive self-talk and think positively) as well as engage in fun, self-esteem building activities. The child should be encouraged to use positive self-talk (e.g., "I'm trying hard and this is great") and learn to look toward the positives, and it may be beneficial to have the child and parent monitor the child's success in using positives, by recording these achievements on a "Being Positive Chart" or on another type of self-monitoring form. Parents may need to learn to be less critical of their youngster and, if depression is "running in the family," then referral of parents for their own therapy may be an essential adjunct to child therapy.

Medications

If the child is taking medication, then the counselor needs to discuss child progress regularly with the pediatrician or psychiatrist who is monitoring medication. Parents and children also need a thorough education about appropriate use of the medications and about whether more negative mood states or changes can occur during the first few weeks or months that the child is taking the medication.

Pharmacotherapy is used to treat childhood depression. Yet, conflicting evidence exists as to whether medications are effective and appropriate to use among children. Selective serotonin reuptake inhibitors, including fluoxetine (or Prozac), have been evaluated in randomized, double-blind, placebo-controlled trial and show significant improvement in depression (Emslie et al., 1997; Emslie, Heiligenstein, & Wagner, 2002). A randomized, double-blind, placebo-controlled trial is a very well-controlled research study that provides some additional confidence in the findings about the effectiveness of a medication. A randomized trial means that each participant has an equal chance of being assigned (at random, often using a random selection chart) to either the treatment or the wait-list control group. A placebo-controlled trial is one where a group of participants might receive a "sugar pill" or a pill to take that does not have any medication. If the children who were taking a placebo medication improved, then it might be that the idea of taking medication improved the child's condition. A double-blind trial is one in which neither the participants in the study nor the research assistants who are collecting data on participant progress know which condition that the participant has been assigned to. Thus, the research assistants and the participants do not know whether a participant is in the treatment or control group. This type of study allows the researcher to make very firm conclusions that if the medication group shows improvement the result is really probably due to the medication and no other factors. Medications have been noted as highly effective in combination with psychotherapy. Health educators who work with children who are depressed can learn from experts about medication adherence and childhood depression from child psychiatrists.

Psychosocial and Emotional Functioning

Depression can impact psychosocial and emotional functioning in children. A study conducted by Fergusson and Woodward (2002) found that social background, familial, and individual factors influenced depression including socioeconomic status (lower family income), mothers with educational underachievement, sexual abuse, parental change, and higher rates of deviant peers. These factors were related to higher levels of sadness in children. Family factors, such as family discord and parental depression, influence the occurrence and maintenance of depression in children (Pilowsky et al., 2006). Children with depressive disorders may have inhibited emotional, cognitive, and social skills that interfere with their family and personal relationships (Birmaher et al., 1996; Lewinsohn et al., 2003). Regarding school, a child's academic performance may be hindered by depression (Owens, Stevenson, Hadwin, & Norgate, 2012). Children who feel disconnected from school tend to report higher depressive symptoms (Millings, Buck, Montgomery, Spears, & Stallard, 2012). Children who experience depression are at increased risk of negative outcomes during late adolescence and young adulthood including later depression, anxiety disorders, nicotine and substance dependence, suicidal behavior, academic failure, and unemployment (Fergusson & Woodward, 2002).

Interventions for Children with Depression and their Caregivers

This section gives an overview of common interventions for children with depression. A recent study conducted by Zhou et al. (2015) reviewed 52 critical studies in the area and found that cognitive-behavioral therapy (CBT) was effective in reducing symptoms of depression both after treatment had ended and at a follow-up assessment a few months later. Cognitive-behavioral therapy (CBT), a type of psychotherapy, is an effective treatment that combines a focus on how a child's thoughts and beliefs influence his/her mood and actions and how a child's actions change behavior patterns. For example, children can change negative thoughts about themselves into more positive ones and reward themselves when they accomplish things, which can improve their mood. Parents can also reward children's accomplishments and be role models for a positive outlook on events that occur within the family. Prior research has found that CBT is efficacious for treatment of children with depression (Arnberg & Ost, 2014; Compton et al., 2004).

A computerized CBT program called, "Stressbusters," has been proven effective for children with mild to moderate depression (Abeles et al., 2009; Smith et al., 2015). Stressbusters is a computer-based program that delivers intervention components via interactive multimedia such as videos and animations. Stressbusters components include education about depression and its treatment, behavioral activation (i.e., applying behavioral techniques learned during programming), identifying and changing negative thoughts, improving social skills and problem-solving skills, as well as education about ways to prevent relapse or recurrence of depressed feelings. Each session of this CBT encompasses reports on the child's current mood and homework, an introduction to the session topic, watching a video of a depressed young actor implementing a treatment technique, and the child designing their own individualized homework based on the treatment technique. Smith et al. (2015) study conducted among 112 children with significant symptoms of depression found improvements in depressive symptoms according to child self-report. These improvements were similar for boys and girls, and the gains they made were maintained at the 3- and 6-month follow-up assessments. A preceding study conducted by Abeles et al. (2009) using the same treatment techniques also found significant improvement in depressive symptoms for children, and these improvements in child functioning were maintained at a follow-up assessment.

A cognitive-behavioral depression prevention program called the Penn Resiliency Program has been effective in reducing depressive symptoms in children who attend middle school (Gillham et al., 2007). This program is a group intervention that teaches children cognitive-behavioral and problem-solving skills. During the program, students learn about the following topics: (1) the association between feelings, beliefs, and behaviors, (2) cognitive styles (e.g., how to change from a more pessimistic to a more positive outlook), and (3) cognitive restructuring skills (e.g., challenging negative thinking). Children also learn a range of coping and problem-solving techniques including how to be assertive, make decisions, negotiate, and relax. Findings from the Gillham et al. (2007) study revealed that schools are an opportune setting to implement the Penn Resiliency Program and teach depression prevention skills. Health educators can help to deliver this beneficial program in the schools.

Roles for Health Educators and Mental Health Professionals

Health educators can initiate prevention programs for children with depression at the primary, secondary, and tertiary level. Primary prevention is before the disease occurs and is designed to prevent the disease or condition via risk reduction (Friis, 2010). An example of primary prevention is targeting children at high risk for developing depression and teaching them healthy behaviors to prevent the onset of depression. Secondary prevention is during the progression of the disease and attempts to identify the disease at its earliest stage via screening procedures and early interventions (Friis, 2010). An example of secondary prevention is a child being screened for depression by a health professional. Tertiary prevention is during later stages of the disease and attempts to reduce the consequences of a disease after the disease has developed to eliminate or at least delay complications and disability associated with the disease (Friis, 2010). An example of tertiary prevention is facilitating a group intervention for children with a depressive disorder and teaching them how to control their depression through stress management techniques and enhancing their communication and problem-solving skills.

Health educators should seek to incorporate factors inherent within a child and the child's family, school, and community within these programs. For example, in primary prevention efforts, health educators can train an audience of school personnel, community professionals, family members, and children on the signs and symptoms of depression. Early recognition of depression increases the likelihood of effective treatment. At the secondary prevention level, health educators can focus on students with risk factors and psychosocial issues that increase their susceptibility to depression. Health educators can teach children how to increase mood via positive self-talk . For example, if a student says "I cannot do this" or "I hate when this happens," health educators can teach them to change these negative statements into positive statements such as "I will do the best I can on this" or "I have dealt with this before and know how to deal with this." At the tertiary level of prevention programming, health educators can support and enhance the psychosocial functioning of students who have depression. Some strategies health educators can use in this type of programming include teaching stress management skills, social skills, communication skills, problem-solving skills, and how to handle negative thoughts. For example, as previously noted, familial conflict influences depression. By teaching children communication and problem-solving skills, health educators can help to eliminate or greatly reduce complications associated with depression. Health educators can help build depressed children's skills by asking children to define the problem, brainstorm for solutions, decide on how to communicate the solution, and details on how to move forward with the agreed upon solution in a healthy way without using negative behaviors (e.g., putting down the other person, accusing the other person). Health educators can play a key role in identifying depression in children and referring them for evaluation and treatment.

Case Study

Marvin is an 11-year-old boy. He is African-American and resides with his maternal grandmother. He has a younger sister and brother, who turn to him for guidance, support, and comfort. Two years ago, his mother died in a car accident. His father had died around the time when the youngest child in the family, his sister, was born. Therefore, he did not really know his father. For the past year, Marvin has been sleeping more than usual, in terms of his typical sleeping habits, which used to be about 9 h per night. He also has been taking naps, which is not something he used to do, even as a younger child. He has not been eating well and has been losing weight. He has been complaining of feeling like, "nothing is really fun right now." He stopped going outside to play with his friends in the neighborhood. Often, he is alone in his room listening to music. Moreover, his grades have dropped in school and he is not regularly completing his homework assignments. He is very quiet in the classroom and often appears to stare into space and be daydreaming. His grandmother has been very worried about his functioning and reports that, "Marvin is just not himself." She brought the aforementioned symptoms to the doctor's attention at Marvin's yearly physical exam about a month ago. Marvin's pediatrician wondered about possible depression and made a referral to the local mental health clinic, in order for Marvin to receive an evaluation of his emotional functioning.

Marvin's grandmother attended the first session with the counselor, where she responded to many background questions. She described the symptoms above (e.g., sleeping more, appetite change, grades dropping, loss of interest in friends and typical activities). After discussing all of these issues, the counselor began to ask her about Marvin's mood and other aspects of his emotional functioning. Marvin's grandmother described his mood as "blue most of the time." She described sadness, but then qualified this by saying, "He's not terribly sad, just down in the dumps all the time this past year." She mentioned that Marvin does not care about his appearance and was not as interested in interacting with peers as he used to be.

Marvin's grandmother mentioned that he was being a, "wonderful big brother, always supporting and caring for his younger brother and sister." She worried, however, that all his care-taking of his siblings was leaving Marvin little room to be a child and take care of himself. Upon further questioning, Marvin's grandmother described his thought processes as clear. That is, Marvin was not experiencing any types of hallucinations, where he had sensory experiences that were not normal, or delusions, thinking things that were not realistic. Further questioning with his grandmother revealed that his thought processes were normal (or clear) and that he was not experiencing any type of symptoms that might indicate a psychotic episode, which might consist of hallucinations or delusions. Marvin was not exhibiting obsessive thoughts or excessive worry, where he tended to review the same type of thoughts and review his worries over and over through negative self-talk. Hence, his cognitive functioning was fairly normal. It was just that, as his grandmother stated, "He's down all the time. He is still able to go to school and function. He's just 'blue' and not my Marvin."

The counselor then had an interview with Marvin. Marvin was intelligent and it was evident that his thinking processes were clear. He was sad and said, "I've been really down for the last year." Upon further questioning, Marvin denied ever feeling suicidal. He never thought of harming himself and would never try because, "My brothers and sisters need me, besides, people shouldn't think like that, life is worth it." He did say he has been feeling sad because he cannot get over the loss of his mother. He mentioned that he did not have a father as a mentor, friend, and role model. He reported that he loves his brother and sister, but wished he could play with them and have fun with them rather than, "telling them what to do all the time." Marvin confirmed that he was feeling tired "all the time." He said that all food, "tastes the same and I just don't like eating like I used to."

Marvin mentioned that he gets along well with other boys his age and has friends, but had not felt like he wanted to interact with peers. He reported that he needed to be alone most of the time. Marvin felt that his sad feelings would not be acceptable to the other boys, who tended to like to laugh and joke with each other. The counselor asked some other questions, about Marvin's likes, dislikes, how he was getting along with his grandmother, how school was going, and his goals for the future. It was noteworthy that Marvin did not see ahead into the future saying, "Oh, I do not think much of what I can be. I am just making it every day to try to deal with it all." Marvin's other responses indicated he still had interests (e.g., football and video games) and that he felt he had a good and strong relationship with his grandmother. He felt that his grandmother was available to talk with him about things, but he felt he could not talk with her, because she was so sad that her daughter had passed away.

After meeting with Marvin, the counselor met with his grandmother alone. The counselor talked with Marvin's grandmother about a possible diagnosis for Marvin, discussing with her the impact of a long-standing, milder grade of depression, such as Marvin was experiencing. The counselor explained that this long-standing depression was called persistent depressive disorder or dysthymic disorder, and although it was not as severe as a more major depression it could have a very negative impact on a child's functioning. The counselor recommended that Marvin participate in weekly therapy so that he could learn strategies to improve his mood and have a place to discuss his feelings. The counselor also mentioned that Marvin might need a place to work through grief related to the loss of his mother and father. Marvin's grandmother agreed that Marvin would need counseling and that the current counselor could discuss Marvin's diagnosis with him.

The counselor next met with Marvin and explained his symptoms and diagnosis. Then, the counselor talked with Marvin about the value of counseling in terms of having a place to discuss his feelings and learn strategies to work through his sad feelings. The counselor also discussed the fact that Marvin might need a place to talk about his feelings related to his mother's and father's deaths. Marvin replied that he might benefit from having someone to talk to, because his grandmother was always too sad when he attempted to discuss his mother's death with her. The counselor asked Marvin if he would like to participate in counseling at his school. Marvin said that he would not want to do this, because he would not want his friends to see him going to see a counselor, because they deal with "crazy people." He felt he did not want other children to know that he needed help. He said that he might be willing to talk to another counselor at the mental health center. He would be willing to try one or two visits to see if he could talk to a counselor in this setting. The counselor asked Marvin's grandmother if Marvin could be seen at the clinic. His grandmother had been worried about having the time and energy to drive Marvin to counseling. After she learned that Marvin was embarrassed to be seen at the school, she agreed to bring him to the mental health clinic. She scheduled an appointment with the counselor they were speaking with.

Summary

This chapter defined different types of depressive disorders common in children. Interventions can be successful in treating childhood depression, but recurrence of these disorders can persist throughout a child's life. Increasing children's understanding of symptoms of depression may help them to reach out for help from professionals. Psychotherapy, including CBT, may be effective in treating childhood depression. Children can use positive imagery and visualize happy images when they feel sad or blue and can also learn stress reduction techniques including controlled breathing and progressive muscle relaxation. Including education and parent and family sessions may increase the effectiveness of this treatment. Computer-based CBT has also been effective and should be further explored for children, especially due to potential problems with access to treatment and increased use of the Internet. Finally, health educators can assist with prevention programming at the primary, secondary, and tertiary level by including families, schools, and the community by increasing knowledge awareness of depression and its treatment.

Exercises/Review Questions

1. Define major depressive disorder.
2. Define some treatments that might be used in psychotherapy.
3. Define primary prevention, secondary prevention, and tertiary prevention and provide examples of each level of prevention.
4. The counselor told Marvin's grandmother that he may have a dysthymic disorder diagnosis. Which symptoms were being exhibited that informed the counselor's diagnosis of a dysthymic disorder?
5. Do you believe Marvin's grandmother was depressed? If yes, how would you recommend treatment to her?
6. Marvin told the counselor he did not want to receive counseling at school due to the stigma of being potentially labeled as "crazy" by his peers. As a health educator, what ideas do you have to help change children's negative views of mental health problems?

Key Concepts

Major depressive disorder
Disruptive mood dysregulation disorder
Persistent depressive disorder
Anhedonia
Suicidal ideation
Psychotherapy
Positive self-statements
Positive imagery
Somatic complaints
Cognitive-behavioral therapy
Stressbusters program
Primary prevention
Secondary prevention
Tertiary prevention

References

Abeles, P., Verduyn, C., Robinson, A., Smith, P., Yule, W., & Proudfoot, J. (2009). Computerized CBT for adolescent depression ("Stressbusters") and its initial evaluation through an extended case series. *Behavioural and Cognitive Psychotherapy, 37*(2), 151–165. doi:10.1017/S1352465808005067.

Alegría, M., Chatterji, P., Wells, K., Cao, Z., Chen, C., Takeuchi, D., … Meng, X. (2008). Disparity in depression treatment among racial and ethnic minority populations in the United States. *Psychiatric Services, 59*(11), 1264–1272. doi: 10.1176/appi.ps.59.11.1264.

American Psychiatric Association. (2013). *Diagnostic and statistical manual of mental disorders: DSM-V* (5th ed.). Washington, DC: American Psychiatric Publishing.

Angold, A., & Costello, E. J. (2000). The child and adolescent psychiatric assessment (CAPA). *Journal of the American Academy of Child & Adolescent Psychiatry, 39*(1), 39–48. doi:10.1097/00004583-200001000-00015.

Angold, A., & Costello, E. J. (2006). Puberty and depression. *Child and Adolescent Psychiatric Clinics of North America, 15*(4), 919–937.

Angold, A., Costello, E. J., & Erkanli, A. (1999). Comorbidity. *Journal of Child Psychology and Psychiatry, 40*(1), 57–87. doi:10.1111/1469-7610.00424.

Arnberg, A., & Ost, L. (2014). CBT for children with depressive symptoms: A meta-analysis. *Cognitive Behaviour Therapy, 43*(4), 275–288.

Avenevoli, S., Stolar, M., Li, J., Dierker, L., & Ries Merikangas, K. (2001). Comorbidity of depression in children and adolescents: Models and evidence from a prospective high-risk family study. *Biological Psychiatry, 49*(12), 1071–1081. doi:10.1016/S0006-3223(01)01142-8.

Axelson, D. A., & Birmaher, B. (2001). Relation between anxiety and depressive disorders in childhood and adolescence. *Depression and Anxiety, 14*(2), 67–78. doi:10.1002/da.1048.

Birmaher, B., Ryan, N. D., Williamson, D. E., Brent, D. A., Kaufman, J., Dahl, R. E., ... Nelson, B. (1996). Childhood and adolescent depression: A review of the past 10 years. Part I. *Journal of the American Academy of Child & Adolescent Psychiatry, 35*(11), 1427–1439. doi: 10.1097/00004583-199611000-00011.

Caspi, A., Braithwaite, A., Poulton, R., Sugden, K., Moffitt, T. E., Taylor, A., ... Martin, J. (2003). Influence of life stress on depression: Moderation by a polymorphism in the 5-HTT gene. *Science, 301*(5631), 386–389. doi: 10.1126/science.1083968.

Compton, S. N., March, J. S., Brent, D., Albano, A. M., Weersing, V. R., & Curry, J. (2004). Cognitive-behavioral psychotherapy for anxiety and depressive disorders in children and adolescents: An evidence-based medicine review. *Journal of the American Academy of Child & Adolescent Psychiatry, 43*(8), 930–959. doi:10.1097/01.chi.0000127589.57468.bf.

Cooper, P., & Goodyer, I. (1993). A community study of depression in adolescent girls. I: Estimates of symptom and syndrome prevalence. *The British Journal of Psychiatry, 163*(3), 369–374. doi:10.1192/bjp.163.3.369.

Costello, E. J., Erkanli, A., & Angold, A. (2006). Is there an epidemic of child or adolescent depression? *Journal of Child Psychology and Psychiatry, 47*(12), 1263–1271. doi:10.1111/j.1469-7610.2006.01682.x.

Costello, E. J., Lewinsohn, P. M., Hellander, M., Hoagwood, K., Koretz, D. S., Nelson, C. A., ... Kaufman, J. (2002). Development and natural history of mood disorders. *Biological Psychiatry, 52*(6), 529–542. doi: 10.1016/S0006-3223(02)01372-0.

Cummings, J. R., & Druss, B. G. (2011). Racial/ethnic differences in mental health service use among adolescents with major depression. *Journal of the American Academy of Child & Adolescent Psychiatry, 50*(2), 160–170. doi:10.1016/j.jaac.2010.11.004.

Dougherty, L. R., Smith, V. C., Bufferd, S. J., Carlson, G. A., Stringaris, A., Leibenluft, E., & Klein, D. N. (2014). DSM-5 disruptive mood dysregulation disorder: Correlates and predictors in young children. *Psychological Medicine, 44*(11), 2339–2350. doi: 10.1017/S0033291713003115.

Egger, H. L., & Angold, A. (2006). Common emotional and behavioral disorders in preschool children: Presentation, nosology, and epidemiology. *Journal of Child Psychology and Psychiatry, and Allied Disciplines, 47*(3/4), 313–337.

Emslie, G. J., Bush, A. J., Weinberg, W. A., Kowactch, B. A., Hughes, C. W., Carmody, T., & Rintelmann, J. (1997). A double-blind, randomized, placebo-controlled trial of fluoxetine in children and adolescents with depression. *Archives of General Psychiatry, 54*(11), 1031–1037. doi: 10.1001/archpsyc.1997.01830230069010.

Emslie, G. J., Heiligenstein, J. H., & Wagner, K. D. (2002). Fluoxetine for acute treatment of depression in children and adolescents: A placebo-controlled, randomized clinical trial. *Journal of the American Academy of Child and Adolescent Psychiatry, 41*(10), 1205–1215.

Fergusson, D. M., & Woodward, L. J. (2002). Mental health, educational, and social role outcomes of adolescents with depression. *Archives of General Psychiatry, 59*(3), 225–231. doi:10.1001/archpsyc.59.3.225.

Field, L. F., Seligman, L., & Albrecht, A. (2008). Mood disorders in children and adolescents. In R. R. Erk (Ed.), *Counseling treatment for children and adolescents with DSM-IV-TR disorders* (2nd ed., pp. 253–293). Upper Saddle River, NJ: Pearson Education.

Fombonne, E., Wostear, G., Cooper, V., Harrington, R., & Rutter, M. (2001). The Maudsley long-term follow-up of child and adolescent depression: 1. Psychiatric outcomes in adulthood. *The British Journal of Psychiatry, 179*(3), 210–217. doi:10.1192/bjp.179.3.210.

Friis, R. H. (2010). *Epidemiology 101*. Burlington, MA: Jones & Bartlett Learning.

Gillham, J. E., Gallop, R., Seligman, M. E. P., Reivich, K. J., Freres, D. R., Chaplin, T. M., … Lascher, M. (2007). School-based prevention of depressive symptoms: A randomized controlled study of the effectiveness and specificity of the penn resiliency program. *Journal of Consulting and Clinical Psychology, 75*(1), 9–19. doi: 10.1037/0022-006X.75.1.9.

Goodman, E., Huang, B., Wade, T. J., & Kahn, R. S. (2003). A multilevel analysis of the relation of socioeconomic status to adolescent depressive symptoms: Does school context matter? *Journal of Pediatrics, 143*(4), 451–456. doi:10.1067/S0022-3476(03)00456-6.

Hammen, C., Brennan, P. A., Keenan-Miller, D., Hazel, N. A., & Najman, J. M. (2010). Chronic and acute stress, gender, and serotonin transporter gene-environment interactions predicting depression symptoms in youth. *Journal of Child Psychology and Psychiatry, 51*(2), 180–187. doi:10.1111/j.1469-7610.2009.02177.x.

Hammen, C., Shih, J., Altman, T., & Brennan, P. A. (2003). Interpersonal impairment and the prediction of depressive symptoms in adolescent children of depressed and nondepressed mothers. *Journal of the American Academy of Child & Adolescent Psychiatry, 42*(5), 571–577. doi:10.1097/01.CHI.0000046829.95464.E5.

Kaufman, J., Martin, A., King, R. A., & Charney, D. (2001). Are child-, adolescent-, and adult-onset depression one and the same disorder? *Biological Psychiatry, 49*(12), 980–1001. doi:10.1016/S0006-3223(01)01127-1.

Kendler, K. S., Kuhn, J. W., Vittum, J., Prescott, C. A., & Riley, B. (2005). The interaction of stressful life events and a serotonin transporter polymorphism in the prediction of episodes of major depression: A replication. *Archives of General Psychiatry, 62*(5), 529–535. doi:10.1001/archpsyc.62.5.529.

Kessler, R. C., Avenevoli, S., & Ries Merikangas, K. (2001). Mood disorders in children and adolescents: An epidemiologic perspective. *Biological Psychiatry, 49*(12), 1002–1014. doi:10.1016/S0006-3223(01)01129-5.

Kessler, R. C., McGonagle, K. A., Swartz, M., Blazer, D. G., & Nelson, C. B. (1993). Sex and depression in the national comorbidity survey I: Lifetime prevalence, chronicity and recurrence. *Journal of Affective Disorders, 29*(2), 85–96. doi:10.1016/0165-0327(93)90026-G.

Kim-Cohen, J., Caspi, A., Moffitt, T. E., Harrington, H., Mine, B. J., & Poulton, R. (2003). Prior juvenile diagnoses in adults with mental disorder: Developmental follow-back of a prospective-longitudinal cohort. *Archives of General Psychiatry, 60*(7), 709–717. doi:10.1001/archpsyc.60.7.709.

Klein, D. N., Dougherty, L. R., & Olino, T. M. (2005). Toward guidelines for evidence-based assessment of depression in children and adolescents. *Journal of Clinical Child & Adolescent Psychology, 34*(3), 412–432. doi:10.1207/s15374424jccp3403_3.

Kovacs, A., Akiskal, S., Gatsonis, C., & Parrone, P. L. (1994). Childhood-onset dysthymic disorder: Clinical features and prospective naturalistic outcome. *Archives of General Psychiatry, 51*(5), 365–374. doi:10.1001/archpsyc.1994.03950050025003.

Kubik, M. Y., Lytle, L. A., Birnbaum, A. S., Murray, D. M., & Perry, C. L. (2003). Prevalence and correlates of depressive symptoms in young adolescents. *American Journal of Health Behavior, 27*(5), 546–553.

Leech, S. L., Larkby, C. A., Day, N. L., & Day, R. (2006). Predictors and correlates of high levels of depression and anxiety symptoms among children at age 10. *Journal of the American Academy of Child & Adolescent Psychiatry, 45*(2), 223–230. doi:10.1097/01.chi.0000184930.18552.4d.

Lewinsohn, P. M., Rohde, P., Seeley, J. R., Klein, D. N., & Gotlib, I. H. (2003). Psychosocial functioning of young adults who have experienced and recovered from major depressive disorder during adolescence. *Journal of Abnormal Psychology, 112*(3), 353–363. doi:10.1037/0021-843X.112.3.353.

Lewinsohn, P. M., Rohde, P., Seeley, J. R., & Hops, H. (1991). Comorbidity of unipolar depression: I. major depression with dysthymia. *Journal of Abnormal Psychology, 100*(2), 205–213. doi:10.1037/0021-843X.100.2.205.

Lewinsohn, P. M., Rohde, P., & Seeley, J. R. (1998). Major depressive disorder in older adolescents. *Clinical Psychology Review, 18*(7), 765–794. doi:10.1016/S0272-7358(98)00010-5.

Lorant, V., Deliège, D., Eaton, W., Robert, A., Philippot, P., & Ansseau, M. (2003). Socioeconomic inequalities in depression: A meta-analysis. *American Journal of Epidemiology, 157*(2), 98–112. doi:10.1093/aje/kwf182.

Luby, J. L., Heffelfinger, A. K., & Mrakotsky, C. (2003). The clinical picture of depression in preschool children. *Journal of the American Academy of Child and Adolescent Psychiatry, 42*(3), 340–348.

McLaughlin, C. L., & Christner, R. W. (2012). Depression: School-based cognitive-behavioral interventions. In R. B. Mennuti, R. W. Christner, & A. Freeman (Eds.), *Cognitive-behavioral interventions in educational settings: A handbook for practice* (2nd ed., pp. 215–238). New York, NY: Routledge: A Taylor and Francis Group.

Millings, A., Buck, R., Montgomery, A., Spears, M., & Stallard, P. (2012). School connectedness, peer attachment, and self-esteem as predictors of adolescent depression. *Journal of Adolescence, 35*(4), 1061–1067. doi:10.1016/j.adolescence.2012.02.015.

Nomura, Y., Wickramaratne, P. J., Warner, V., Mufson, L., & Weissman, M. M. (2002). Family discord, parental depression, and psychopathology in offspring: Ten-year follow-up. *Journal of the American Academy of Child & Adolescent Psychiatry, 41*(4), 402–409. doi:10.1097/00004583-200204000-00012.

Owens, M., Stevenson, J., Hadwin, J. A., & Norgate, R. (2012). Anxiety and depression in academic performance: An exploration of the mediating factors of worry and working memory. *School Psychology International, 33*(4), 433–449.

Pilowsky, D. J., Wickramaratne, P., Nomura, Y., & Weissman, M. M. (2006). Family discord, parental depression, and psychopathology in offspring: 20-year follow-up. *Journal of the American Academy of Child & Adolescent Psychiatry, 45*(4), 452–460. doi:10.1097/01.chi.0000198592.23078.8d.

Pine, D. S., Cohen, P., Johnson, J. G., & Brook, J. S. (2002). Adolescent life events as predictors of adult depression. *Journal of Affective Disorders, 68*(1), 49–57. doi:10.1016/S0165-0327(00)00331-1.

Poznanski, E. O., & Mokros, H. B. (1999). *Children depression rating scale—Revised (CDRS-R)*. Los Angeles, CA: Western Psychological Services.

Smith, P., Verduyn, C., Yule, W., Scott, R., Eshkevari, E., Jatta, F., … Proudfoot, J. (2015). Computerised CBT for depressed adolescents: Randomised controlled trial. *Behaviour Research and Therapy, 73*, 104–110. doi: 10.1016/j.brat.2015.07.009.

Substance Abuse and Mental Health Services Administration. (2014). *Results from the 2013 national survey on drug use and health: Summary of national findings* (NSDUH Series H-48, HHS Publication No. (SMA) 14-4863 ed.). Rockville, MD: Substance Abuse and Mental Health Services Administration.

Tracy, M., Zimmerman, F. J., Galea, S., McCauley, E., & Stoep, A. V. (2008). What explains the relation between family poverty and childhood depressive symptoms? *Journal of Psychiatric Research, 42*(14), 1163–1175. doi:10.1016/j.jpsychires.2008.01.011.

Weissman, M. M., Wickramaratne, P., Nomura, Y., Warner, V., Verdeli, H., Pilowsky, D. J., … Bruder, G. (2005). Families at high and low risk for depression: A 3-generation study. *Archives of General Psychiatry, 62*(1), 29–36. doi: 10.1001/archpsyc.62.1.29.

World Health Organization. (2015). *International classification of mental and behavioral disorders, 10th revision (ICD-10)*. Geneva, Switzerland: World Health Organization.

Zhou, X., Michael, K. D., Zhang, Y., Weisz, J. R., Xie, P., Hetrick, S. E., … Liu, Y. (2015). Comparative efficacy and acceptability of psychotherapies for depression in children and adolescents: A systematic review and network meta-analysis. *World Psychiatry, 14*(2), 207–222. doi: 10.1002/wps.20217.

Chapter 9
Conduct Problems

Diagnosis

Blair, Leibenluft, and Pine (2014) referred to conduct problems as "...a pattern of repetitive rule-breaking behavior, aggression, and disregard for others" (p. 2207). It is these types of behaviors, when they reach a consistent pattern that interferes with a child's daily functioning, that are the focus of this chapter. Kazdin (1997) defined conduct disorder in this manner,

"The overarching feature of conduct disorder is a persistent pattern of behavior in which the rights of others and age-appropriate social norms are violated. Isolated acts of physical aggression, destruction of property, stealing and fire setting are sufficiently severe to warrant concern and attention in their own right. Although these behaviors may occur in isolation, several of these are likely to appear together as a constellation or syndrome and form the basis of a clinical diagnosis" (p. 162).

In the Diagnostic and Statistical Manual of Mental Disorders (American Psychiatric Association, 2013), conduct problems are in a section entitled, "Disruptive, Impulse Control, and Conduct Disorders (CD)." According to the experts who developed this section of the manual these conditions involve, "... problems in the self-control of emotions and behaviors" (p. 461). These self-control problems are unique in that they, "...violate the rights of others (e.g., aggression, destruction of property) and/or that bring the individual into significant conflict with societal norms or authority figures" (p. 461).

Children who are diagnosed with CD are likely to have other diagnoses. For example, Kazdin (1997) reported that over 80 % of children met the criteria for CD and Oppositional Defiant Disorder (ODD). Many children with CD may be diagnosed with Attention-Deficit Hyperactivity Disorder (Blair, Leibenluft, & Pine, 2014; Kim-Cohen et al., 2005). Children with CD may be diagnosed with co-occurring learning problems, such as reading and/or math disorders. According to the DSM-5 (American Psychiatric Association, 2013), children with CD show at

© Springer International Publishing Switzerland 2016
L. Nabors, *Medical and Mental Health During Childhood*, Springer
Series on Child and Family Studies, DOI 10.1007/978-3-319-31117-3_9

least one symptom indicating aggression toward animals or people, destruction of property, lying or theft, and serious rule violations (e.g., truant from school, runs away from home) before 10 years of age. Children may also have limited empathy and be callous. They can lack remorse or guilt related to violating social norms or the rights of others. They may display very little emotion to other people, which is termed shallow or deficient affect. The essential feature of CD is violating the rights of others or social rules persistently, in such a manner to impair child functioning. CD can occur as early as the preschool years, but is most commonly manifested in middle childhood and early adolescence.

Oppositional Defiant Disorder. A relatively milder version of conduct problems is ODD. Criteria for ODD include having a frequent and stable pattern of "…angry/ irritable mood, argumentative/defiant behavior, or vindictiveness lasting at least 6 months" (p. 462, American Psychiatric Association, 2013). The behaviors associated with ODD need to interfere with the individual's functioning and cause distress to the individual and others in his or her life. The diagnosis is applicable to children as young as 5 years of age. If the symptoms are in a mild range, they may occur only at home. The behaviors also may be more frequent with adults and peers that the child knows fairly well, and thus the symptoms may not always be directly observable in the office or clinical setting. Symptoms can be in the range of mild (symptoms present in one setting), moderate (symptoms present in two settings), and severe (symptoms are present in three or more settings). Although some children with oppositional behaviors develop significant problems to merit a disorder of CD, not all children with ODD follow a progression to the development of a diagnosis of CD. However, although many children with ODD can develop normally, they are at greater risk for developing other mental health problems, including internalizing problems such as anxiety or depression.

Other Externalizing Behaviors. It is beneficial to explain other externalizing behavior problems that may be diagnosed in childhood. Intermittent Explosive Disorder can begin in late childhood and involves an inability to control verbal or physical aggression (the physical aggression does not result in damage of property or injury to others; American Psychiatric Association, 2013). The aggressive outbursts occur about twice weekly for at least 3 months and are damaging for the individual displaying the symptoms. Another externalizing problem can be fire-setting or pyromania. This can occur in childhood, but information about this disorder in children is needed. Kleptomania, or impulsive stealing that is not for monetary value, is most often diagnosed in adolescence. There is also a category in the DSM-5 for Other Disruptive, Impulse-Control, and Conduct Disorders for those children with symptoms that do not clearly "fit" the categories for ODD or CD.

The primary focus of this chapter is on ODD and CD. In samples of participating children and parents for research, children with both of these disorders are often grouped together, so conduct problems is a term commonly used throughout this chapter.

Prevalence

"Prevalence rates for CD vary, ranging from 2 to 10%, with a median of 4%" (p. 473, American Psychiatric Association, 2013). Prevalence rates increase into adolescence. Rates of CD are higher among males compared to females. Males with CD are likely to exhibit significant aggression. Females are aggressive as well, but also are thought to have higher rates of lying, truancy, and stealing. The prevalence for ODD is estimated to be about 3–4%. These types of problems are more commonly diagnosed in males than females (1.4–1) in childhood, but this difference becomes more equal in adolescence and adulthood.

Genetic and Environmental Influences

Many experts agree that when children exhibit conduct problems, there is an interaction between genetic and environmental influences such that both factors play a role in determining behaviors (e.g., Silberg, Maes, & Eaves, 2012; Tolan, Dodge, & Rutter, 2013). Genetic factors, which may predispose a child to exhibit conduct problems, include problems with regulation of emotions and poor frustration tolerance. These may be temperamental factors, which have a genetic loading, that impact the development of conduct problems. Children with conduct problems also may have reduced cortisol activity in their brains, lower heart rates, and lower skin reactivity. Differences in prefrontal cortex activity (a part of the brain involved with higher order thinking and regulation of emotions) and the amygdala (associated with memory and emotional reactions) have been noted in children with ODD and CD. (American Psychiatric Association, 2013).

Parenting that is harsh, critical, and inconsistent can also be related to conduct problems in children (Kazdin, 1997; Okado & Bierman, 2015). Tolan et al. (2013) reported that young children who have attachments with parents that are not secure, experience negative parenting (with inconsistent rules and application of consequences for behavior), and experience inconsistent monitoring of their well-being and safety are more likely to experience behavior problems. Moreover, parent–child relationships that do not show warmth and support, but rather hostility and a lack of connectedness with others may be related to difficulties in functioning. A lack of warmth and hostility in families can be significant in children with CD. In fact, experts for the DSM-5 reported that a host of family risk factors for CD include but are not limited to, "parental rejection and neglect, harsh discipline, physical or sexual abuse, lack of supervision, early institutional living, frequent changes of caregivers, etc." (American Psychiatric Association, 2013, p. 473). Children with CD can grow up to have significant problems, including problems with the criminal justice system and issues with substance use and addictive disorders. There is a chance that children with CD can grow up to display Antisocial Personality Disorder, but this is not a given (i.e., not a certain outcome) if a child is diagnosed with CD. Antisocial Personality Disorder has been considered sociopathy or psychopathy, which is distinguished by a lack of regard for rights of others and social rules. In the current diagnostic manual, Antisocial Personality Disorder is defined, in part, as a, "persistent pattern of disregard for the and violation of the rights of others, occurring since age 15 years…" (American Psychiatric Association, 2013, p. 659).

Impact on Children

Wu et al. (2015) highlighted two features of conduct problems, including consistent rule-breaking and aggression. Wu et al. (2015) described children with CD as having quick and angry tempers and mentioned that children with conduct problems break rules and do not take responsibility for their negative behaviors. They may tend to blame the victim in situations where one child is aggressive toward another. Wu et al. mentioned that children with conduct problems who exhibit aggression and the other aforementioned problems may have poorer outcomes. They may continue to display aggressive behaviors and a lack of responsiveness to rules and social customs. As one can imagine, conduct problems in children have a significant impact on their lives. These problems cause isolation and are associated with a host of other emotional and behavioral problems. These diagnoses can include internalizing problems, such as bipolar disorder, depression, and anxiety, as well as learning problems, intellectual disability, intermittent explosive disorder, and mood dysregulation. Conduct problems are very commonly diagnosed with Attention-Deficit Hyperactivity Disorder (Andrade & Tannock, 2012). Children with conduct problems have poor social abilities and may not have many friends (Andrade & Tannock, 2012; Olson, Lopez-Duran, Lunkenheimer, Chang, & Sameroff, 2011). Children with CD and ODD can experience isolation. They may have significant difficulty regulating their emotional reactions, which can contribute to difficulties with peers and adults as well (Havighurst et al., 2015). Eisenberg et al. (2005) proposed that children who experience risk for development of conduct problems are more likely to react negatively in emotional situations. They are expressing more negative emotions and reacting more negatively, which can further isolate them. Children with significant conduct problems may be at risk for long-term negative behaviors, such as hostility, aggression, rule-breaking, lying, and stealing. These behaviors may be related to psychiatric problems and a lack of positive relationships with peers and adults. Long-term risk for substance use, psychiatric disorders (including antisocial personality disorder), and poor relationships and school and work adjustment may result (Maughan & Rutter, 2001).

Argument for Subgroups. In a review article, in the *Psychological Bulletin*, Frick, Ray, Thornton, and Kahn (2013) proposed that there is a subgroup of children with conduct problems, who exhibit callous and unemotional traits. Children in this subgroup were at heightened risk for long-term psychosocial problems and problems relating to others. Frick et al. mentioned that those studying conduct problems in children and adolescents need to begin to think about subgroups of children with conduct problems. Groups could be determined by the severity of the problems they exhibited as they aged. Those children with CD and callous and unemotional behaviors were at risk for long-term conduct problems. Children with these traits also exhibited cortical differences—that is differences in gray matter in the brain—in some studies. These cortical differences could also be responsible for some children's "hyporesponsiveness" to emotional stimuli. Hyporesponsiveness means that children are under-responsive to stimulation. They often are taking risks and seeking thrills to gain more stimulation. Frick, Ray, Thornton, and Kahn (2013) further distinguished this subgroup of children as having higher to highest levels of deficits in responding to punishment, insensitive to fear expressed by others, and thrill-seeking. Because children in this subgroup may exhibit these issues when they are very young, they may not develop conscientiousness. Although children with more severe problems could have a more bleak long-term prognosis, Frick et al. (2013) cautioned that positive outcomes could occur for children who were callous and unemotional. They proposed that children with the aforementioned symptoms and more severe externalizing problems needed referral to intensive, long-term intervention programs.

Frick et al. (2013) proposed that there was another group that did not exhibit callousness. Children with conduct problems in this group were likely to feel anxiety and worry over the plight of others. Frick et al. speculated that these children were more likely to have learned to exhibit conduct problems after experiencing harsh and inconsistent caregiving. Youth in this group also might exhibit deficits in verbal abilities. Although more information is needed to determine if subgroups exist, it is evident that those children with more severe symptoms, who do not care for the welfare of others, and who do not respond much to punishment are more likely to experience poor outcomes.

Assessment

There are several questions to ask to determine whether children and parents endorse symptoms of CD. Questions to ask include: (1) I take/steal things that don't belong to me, (2) I tell lies, (3) I fight and hit other children a lot, (4) I start fires, (5) I hit and yell at Mommy and Daddy, (6) I like to break rules, (7) I break or ruin other kids' and my family's things, and (8) I hurt animals (Kim-Cohen et al., 2005). Duncombe, Havinghurst, Holland, and Frankling (2012) developed a screening assessment tool for parents and teachers to complete that may assist health educators in making referrals for children who are exhibiting conduct problems. Parents and teachers complete seven questions assessing a child's: (1) attention, (2) fighting and bullying, (3) friendship skills, (4) impulsivity, (5) temper, (6) arguing, and (7) rule-breaking. Children's behaviors are rated on a 5-point scale from "0" never to "4" almost always. Some might argue that self-report could be biased and that health professionals should observe children's behaviors in the home and school settings to have an accurate assessment of the child's functioning. If two informants are used, the types of questions outlined in this assessment section can yield valuable information, because children with severe conduct problems will exhibit the types of behaviors that are "very noticeable."

CD can be assessed in preschool. Early identification may offer opportunities to "turn around" problem behaviors. Questions assessing aggression toward peers and small animals can be useful. Moreover, questions examining impulsivity and the child's ability to follow rules and instructions are appropriate. In addition, learning whether the child can regulate his or her emotional reactions will provide other important information.

Management

There are several treatments that are effective in improving behavioral, social, and emotional functioning of children with conduct problems. For instance, problem-solving training is an effective treatment for children with CD. Children learn step-by-step processes for solving problems, and often use role play, with trained therapists coaching them, to learn how to control angry reactions and solve problems in positive ways. Problem-solving programs usually involve brainstorming to solve problems with "checking" to make sure that the problem-solving approach worked. In order to begin to learn a problem-solving approach, the child and his or her coach (a trained educator or therapist) typically develop two or three acceptable plans to solve a hypothetical social or behavioral problem. Then, they select a best course of action and it is implemented. The child then checks the results of the problem-solving plan to see if it was successful. If the approach was not successful, the child needs to problem-solve again or try another plan. The child needs to implement plan two and again check for its success. Due to their impulsivity and seeing hostility in others, children with conduct problems do not always select a prosocial solution or try to find another solution if their first one did not work. Children with conduct problems may need additional practice, using role plays, to learn problem-solving steps. They may need behavior charts with rewards and contracts, which are monitored by adults with knowledge of children's behavioral goals to ensure that they use problem-solving steps.

Children with CD may benefit from participating in anger management groups or individual counseling (Powell et al., 2011). Therapy goals, in addition to using role plays to learn positive behaviors, may include activities to ensure that children are more aware of their emotions and learn anger management skills. Children with conduct problems may tend to react aggressively and strongly and thus learning their "anger triggers" or cues that signal that they are going to become angry can be very important. Children need to learn their cues for anger and aggressive behaviors, and then need to learn to calm themselves, using relaxation or positive self-talk, and then implement problem-solving skills. Individual therapy sessions or groups are avenues for learning about personal triggers and emotional regulation and problem-solving skills. Children with conduct problems also may need to learn perspective-taking skills, where they practice thinking how the other person may feel and thinking how their actions may influence others. This may be especially important if the child has relatively weaker skills for being empathic and for a child who may be unemotional or callous.

Parent training is another critical component for management of conduct problems in children. Parents may need training because they are inconsistent in their discipline or ineffective in using appropriate behavior management strategies with their child (Patterson & Stouthamer-Loeber, 1984). Webster-Stratton's Incredible Years, for example, is built on a parent-training component where parents watch videos to learn how to use praise and rewards and avoid harsh and critical parenting (Webster-Stratton, Reid, & Hammond, 2004). In training sessions, parents also learn to use appropriate consequences, such as loss of privileges or time-out, if the child is misbehaving. For time-out, a child is placed in a chair for 1 min for each year of age. After a period of quietly sitting (parents are not to talk back and forth with the child while he or she is in time-out), then the child can resume activities. The boredom associated with time-out or withdrawal from doing fun things and from attention is a consequence for the child. Response cost is another term for loss of privileges or loss of being able to participate in a valued activity. A response cost is an alternative to using time-out. A response cost needs to be clearly specified at a time when the child and parent are calm. During this "meeting" the parent can explain the one or two behaviors that will result in a response cost. For example, "if you hit your brother or sister, then you will lose 20 min of computer time." It is important to try not to take all privileges away from the child, because this can be very disheartening and some children may behave badly if all privileges are taken away for long periods of time. Making sure that the punishment is fair, in terms of actually being a cost and ensuring that the penalty is not too stiff, is part of the art of parenting.

Modeling appropriate behaviors through role play activities and when there are "teachable moments" during daily activities is another assignment for parents. Children "learn what they live" and opportunities arise for modeling positive behaviors during daily interactions. Involving children in groups and clubs with positive peer and adult role models can be avenues for finding positive role models for children. Role plays, in which specific prosocial scripts are reviewed, are other ways to "practice" positive social routines with a child. Developing a list of problem situations and then reviewing successful behaviors with a child through role play several times a week are a possible homework assignment for parents working with their child to improve negative behaviors.

Children with conduct problems may have difficulty monitoring the appropriateness of their own behavior. They may need to learn self-monitoring skills and positive self-talk for working out aggressive or negative reactions. The child needs to learn to "watch" or monitor his or her own behavior to ensure that he or she is stopping to think about positive responses. The child needs to talk him- or herself through a series of positive actions and then praise him- or herself for positive behaviors. The child may not do this on his or her own. The parent can be taught to model this behavior for the child and practice it with him or her on a regular basis.

The child also may benefit from having a reward chart where he or she earns stickers, which lead to treats and rewards, for those times that the child engages in self-monitoring. Parents need to ensure that the positive self-talk resulted in a positive outcome. Self-monitoring also can be used to control negative behaviors. Thus, a child can be self-monitoring to praise him- or herself for not behaving negatively toward others. A child is then rewarded for an absence of negative behaviors. Although this can seem like a "bribe" to some parents, it is important to explain that providing a reward for self-control and positive self-talk is a way to show children how important the behavior is to parents and a mechanism to help them pay attention to what they are doing. Rewards can be small, but it is important to ensure that the rewards are meaningful to the child.

Other skills are taught in parent training. Two of these skills are shaping appropriate behaviors and teaching anger management skills (e.g., expressing feelings and learning to control impulsive responding). In shaping of appropriate behaviors, parents are taught to model appropriate behaviors and reward children's approximations (small steps) toward a desired behavior. In terms of friendship skills, a first step might be to teach a child to greet another child. After the child has practiced the behavior, then the parent should praise and reward the child for his or her effort. If the child gains this skill, then a possible next step is to reward a child for learning how to ask to join in play with other children. Another goal might be working with a child to take turns in conversations with others. In a step-by-step process, each goal or task is broken into smaller, more manageable "chunks" of behavior and the child is praised or rewarded for mastery of each step in the chain of behaviors. In the long run, the child is learning better friendship skills, one skill at a time.

Another component of parent training might be teaching contingency contracting with an older child. This is a behavioral contract that "spells out" the desired behavior for a child. The child agrees to exhibit a behavior in return for a privilege or reward. At times the child signs the contract and at other times verbally agrees to the contract. There may often be consequences for misbehavior recorded in the contract. Contingency contracts may work better if they are specific in nature, spelling out the steps of the desired behavior in very clear language. Contingency contracting may be an effective tool if applied consistently without adopting a harsh or punitive attitude toward the child. Consequences need to be used consistently and fairly with children who have conduct problems.

Parents are also taught to spend time in child-directed play with their child, where the child is leading play and parents are supporting the child in his or her activities. This can be called "positive time." This time can help to "break up" the negative cycle of interactions that are occurring between a parent and child. Behavior can move in cycles and parents and children may be trading negative behaviors (Patterson, 1982). Accordingly, it may be child negative behaviors are influencing parent reactions in a negative manner. Although parents may be harsh with the child, it also is the case that the child's own negative behaviors bring out a harsh reaction in the parent. This bidirectional influence could play a role in the negative parent–child relationship cycle. Positive time with the child is on the child's own terms and the parent acts more like a sportscaster, talking about what the child is doing during play. The child selects the activities and as long as the child is not aggressive or hurting people or property, the child continues to direct play and the interaction. The parent's role becomes more positive, rather than directive, during child-directed play sessions. These sessions can be short (10 min per day), but should occur consistently or routinely. Hawes, Price, and Dadds (2014) recommended that children and parents also engage in eye contact. They reported that reciprocal eye contact can promote emotional awareness and awareness of the other person in interactions. Hawes et al. emphasized parent–child engagement as key method for improving emotional connectivity of the child.

Furthermore, it is important to remember that child negative behaviors also can impact how parents react to their child. Thus, it is realistic to think that parent behavior could be influencing the child and child conduct problems could be influencing parent behaviors and this bidirectional influence could also play a role in the development of conduct problems displayed by young children.

Powell et al. (2011) examined teacher training to promote effective child behavior in school settings. With the exception of child-directed play, they recommended many of the principles mentioned in the preceding paragraphs can be applied at school. They recommended providing teacher training in the use of praise and rewards to help children learn positive behaviors and use self-control (e.g., self-control techniques involve breathing, relaxation, and positive self-talk to inhibit aggressive responses). They recommended the use of positive goal-setting with child monitoring (using monitoring charts can be helpful) to assist in teaching the child to monitor his or her own behaviors and begin to learn self-control.

Early intervention, in the preschool years, may prevent behavior problems in later years. Selecting children in the top 5 % of problem behaviors that involve aggression toward others and rule-breaking in the preschool period may yield an appropriate sample for intervention programs that target parent and teacher training in contingency management where adults learn the use of rewards, loss of privileges, and consequences and learn ways to consistently apply rules to help a young child improve his or her behaviors. Teachers and parents also may need to learn how to "tune in" to a child's emotional reactions and teach him or her to regulate emotions and learn routines for solving social and other behavioral problems in positive ways.

Medications

Wu et al. (2015) reviewed pharmacological treatments for conduct problems. The cursory review in this paragraph is very general, and professionals working with children with CD should consult child psychiatrists to learn more about medication management. Wu et al. mentioned several medications that were successful in reducing aggressive behaviors exhibited by children with CD. Antipsychotic medications, such as thioridazine, have reduced aggression. However, these types of medications can cause motor movements and impact motor behaviors. Wu et al. reported that nontraditional antipsychotic medications, like risperidone, can reduce children's aggressive behaviors, without as significant of effects on motor symptoms. Stimulant medications, such as those used to treat Attention-Deficit Hyperactivity Disorder, may also have a positive influence on children's behaviors. Antihypertensive medications, most notably clonidine, have been used to treat children with CD. This drug can have a positive impact on behaviors, but has side effects such as drowsiness, weakness, and constipation. Although medication management is a helpful tool in the treatment of CD, a thorough evaluation of the child's functioning is needed. In the long run, combined medication and behavioral/psychological treatments are frontline interventions for children with CD.

Psychosocial Functioning

Children who have conduct problems can be very aggressive (Okado & Bierman, 2015). Young children who are very aggressive and cannot regulate their mood, especially in terms of reacting in anger or aggressively toward others, may be at risk for conduct problems as they age (Okado & Bierman, 2015). Children with CD can be cruel to peers and adults. They can be described as lacking feelings for others and not caring for the well-being of others (Blair et al., 2014). Children with emotional dysregulation and aggression are likely to face peer rejection and difficulty forming positive social relationships. As mentioned, children with conduct problems may be unemotional (Frick et al., 2013). Hawes, Price, and Dadds (2014) mentioned that callous and unemotional traits (i.e., limited prosocial emotions) are a hallmark feature of this diagnosis. Consequently, children with conduct problems might not respond or respond very minimally to distress in other individuals. They may be overly sensitive to threat in the behavior of others and see aggression and hostility in others' behaviors, even if the behaviors were not intended to be aggressive. This may cause children to quickly respond to events that most would consider as being "neutral" in terms of their meaning in a hostile or aggressive manner. If CD persists from the childhood years, then the youth is at risk for substance abuse problems, truancy, and criminal behaviors (e.g., stealing; Blair et al.).

When CD is left untreated or if the child is unresponsive to treatment, psychiatric problems in adulthood are possible (Hawes et al., 2014). Rouquette et al. (2014) found an association between conduct problems in children involving aggression, oppositional and defiant behavior, hyperactivity, fearfulness and feelings of helplessness and having a diagnosis of CD in adolescence. More research into the link between feelings of helplessness and fear and conduct problems will be needed, because these types of behaviors are not always synonymous with conduct problems in other studies. It may be that overly harsh parenting, a lack of emotional connection with others, and seeing the world as a hostile place lead to feelings of fear and helplessness. These types of feelings could lead to more aggressive behaviors. This idea is speculative, and needs to be explored in future longitudinal studies assessing children's psychological functioning and feelings and reactions over extended periods of time.

There may be a physiological explanation related to the diagnosis of CD, especially in boys. Herpertz et al. (2005) found that autonomic responsiveness to stimuli that might be expected to cause a positive or negative emotional reaction was very low in boys with CD. They concluded that boys with CD were very low in physiological responsiveness (e.g., heart rate) to stimuli that might be expected to cause physiological arousal in children without this diagnosis. If boys with conduct problems are under-reactive and they react less to emotion-provoking stimuli, this may be why they are considered unemotional or callous. Youth who are under-responsive may seek stimulation or tolerate high stimulation experiences at a different level than children with what might be considered a more normal physiological reaction to fear-producing stimuli. This phenomenon needs to be studied in depth as many of the participants had other diagnoses, and studies with girls are needed. However, it provides an intriguing consideration for some of the behaviors displayed by males diagnosed with conduct problems.

Children with conduct problems may attribute hostile intentions to others' behaviors (Powell et al., 2011). Dodge (1980) is one of the first researchers to discuss this hostile attribution bias. In his experiments, Dodge showed that children who were classified as being aggressive were more likely to attribute hostile intentions to another child's behavior in ambiguous situations. This was especially true if the outcome of the ambiguous situation was negative for a character described in the situation. The ideas of a hostile attribution bias became a cornerstone of understanding aggressive behaviors for years. Children with conduct problems are deficient in skills for emotional regulation and understanding emotions in social exchanges, which makes teaching them social problem solving very important.

Parent discipline may be inconsistent and harsh (Kazdin, 1997; Kim-Cohen et al., 2005). Parents can display less warmth (hostile parenting may occur) and more inconsistent levels of punishment, but this pattern of behavior may not directly influence conduct problems (Okado & Bierman, 2015). Furthermore, parents can have a history of psychiatric problems or criminality (Powell et al., 2011). Negative behaviors related to psychiatric instability may also influence an inconsistent parenting style and can be related to attachment difficulties between the parent and child. It may be that parents have no role models for positive parenting skills and learning these skills can help them teach their child how to behave.

Interventions

Several training programs, which involve a parent training component, are reviewed in this section of the chapter. There are many effective training programs for parents, which are combined with child and school interventions. The reader is guided to an expert review by Furlong et al. (2013). This review is a Cochrane Review and these reviews are very useful and typically present information on evidence-based interventions. The interventions presented in this section have a heavy parent-training component and the articles are centered on early intervention. Early intervention, in the preschool years, is recommended by experts (Kim-Cohen et al., 2005).

The Conduct Problems Prevention Research Group (2011) examined outcomes for the Fast Track Intervention. Children at high risk for conduct problems were identified in kindergarten and followed from 3rd through 12th grade. These children were diagnosed with a variety of externalizing disorders including Attention-Deficit Hyperactivity Disorder, ODD, CD, and other externalizing problems (e.g., Disruptive Behavior Disorder). Parents participated in behavior management training (there were also home visits) and children learned problem-solving and social skills (participation in friendship groups). In addition, classroom behavior and academic skills training were provided. Children participating in the intervention have exhibited more positive behaviors and fewer negative behaviors, such as aggressive behaviors. Children who were assigned to treatment were less likely to be diagnosed with CD or ODD over time. These results are important, because they show that the trajectory toward negative and conduct problems can be turned around in a positive direction.

The Incredible Years Program can be used with very young children. This program was developed by Webster-Stratton to treat conduct problems in preschool-age children (e.g., Webster-Stratton et al., 2004). Posthumus, Raaijmakers, Maassen, Van Engeland, and Matthys (2012) provided a summary of the Incredible Years Program (more information is available at http://incredibleyears.com/, accessed January 2, 2016). This program provides parent training through observation and discussion of parent–child interactions presented on videotape. A group leader discusses appropriate parenting practice such as use of praise, rewards, child-directed play (the child directs the play interaction with the parent), limit-setting, handling misbehavior, and how to use positive and consistent guidelines with children. There also is an advanced component to this program which involves more information about communication skills and how to problem-solve. In addition, Webster-Stratton and Reid (2010) mentioned that including a teacher training component as part of the Incredible Years programming can assist in teachers in working with children to use encouragement, incentives (rewards), and support child emotion-regulation, social skills development, and problem-solving skills development in the school setting.

Posthumus, Raaijmakers, Maassen, Van Engeland, and Matthys (2012) examined the effectiveness of the Incredible Years Program with a sample of preschool-age children (4 years) from the Netherlands. Parents met with experts and watched over 200 videotaped interactions of parent–child interactions. There was a control group, but this was not a randomly assigned group. The children also were displaying aggression. Child progress was assessed using parent report on surveys and observations of videotapes of parent–child interactions in the home. Results indicated that parents were less critical (using lower levels of critical statements with their child) after participating in treatment and the results "held" in a 2-year follow-up study. Parent use of praise was improved after the intervention ended; however, this gain was not maintained at the 2-year follow-up assessment. Posthumus et al. reported that parent behavior had a strong impact on children over time for parents who received treatment. Conversely, child behavior did not continue to exert a strong impact on parent behavior. This could be an important finding, because parents could be continuing to positively influence the child and could have acquired skills to help them stop or reduce their critical and harsh reactions to child misbehavior. This could mean that the harsh cycle of negative behaviors between the parent and child was disrupted. Posthumus et al. mentioned that the Incredible Years Program is effective in reducing problem behavior in young children. Thus, the Incredible Years Program had a positive impact, but more research is needed to determine if this program actually helps to prevent CD from developing.

Hutchings et al. (2007) examined the influence of the Incredible Years Program in a large-scale trial in England, with preschoolers. They used parent report of behavioral progress and observations in the home to record child progress in changing disruptive behaviors. Children showed reductions in disruptive and hyperactive behaviors. Parents reported greater competence in their parenting skills. Hutchings et al. recommended that in the future researchers should examine the fidelity with which the program was delivered. This means examining whether the intervention programs was delivered according to the steps outlined in the manual.

Havighurst et al. (2015) examined the effectiveness of an emotion-focused coping program for elementary school-aged children with behavior problems and their caregivers. They intervened with children, in kindergarten through third grade (5–9 years of age), who were in the top 8 % in terms of displaying disruptive behavior problems. Their goal was to teach children appropriate skills before behavior problems strengthened in intensity. They used the Turning In To Kids Program; this program is oriented toward emotions and problem-solving. The Turning In To Kids Program teaches parents to help the child recognize and understand his or her emotional experience and teach the child problem-solving skills. The child learned to regulate his or her emotions and implement appropriate behaviors. There was a child, parent training, and school component. Children learned emotional competence and problem-solved different social situations in small groups. Teachers learned a curriculum that emphasized social problem-solving, self-control, and emotional coping. Parents learned similar skills. Children who participated in the intervention showed improvements in their abilities to understand others' emotions.

Roles for Health Educators

Health educators have varied roles to play in the care of children with conduct problems, depending on their training and their areas of expertise. If the child has more severe problems, then specialized training would probably be needed to provide services. Training in setting limits and safety training (training focusing on keeping the child and professional safe if the child is aggressive) are necessary for those who desire to help children with severe conduct problems on special inpatient units. A long course of treatment with therapeutic aftercare in group home settings may be necessary for children with severe conduct problems. Learning to follow rules, respect others' personal boundaries, and follow rules would be a few of the skills the health educator would need to implement in inpatient and group home settings. The health educator or counselor would benefit from receiving specialty training in parent training programs for children with disruptive and oppositional behaviors. The health educator or counselor would need to gain knowledge about teaching parents how to set limits, give clear instructions, establish and remain consistent about consequences, and use rewards and praise appropriately. Teaching parents about steps for shaping positive behaviors and steps for problem-solving with the child would be important skills to teach parents. When children are younger, working on eye contact could be another component of parent training. The health educator or counselor would need similar knowledge of behavior management skills and teaching social skills and problem-solving when working with teachers and other school staff. Interventions with children who have conduct problems are often intensive and long term. The health educator needs to care for his or her own mental, physical, and spiritual health in order to "go the distance" in terms of continuing with treatment.

Case Study

Larry was an elementary student who was referred to the school mental health counselor for cutting a girl's pigtail with his scissors. His teacher was very upset. She reported that Larry had problems getting along with the other boys and girls. He was frequently in fights with other boys and girls on the playground and in the neighborhood. She also stated that he never completed his homework and tended to make noise and talk with others, disrupting the classroom and making it difficult for the other children to complete their work. He tended to argue with the teacher, which she described as "talking back and being rude and disrespectful to adults." Larry's teacher had been having difficulty reaching his grandmother, who was his legal guardian. His mother was using drugs and the family did not know where she was. There was not information on Larry's father, and Larry had never met him.

The school counselor was able to reach Larry's grandmother for an interview. His grandmother provided consent for the counselor to work with Larry. At her interview, Larry's grandmother appeared distraught and said she was unsure of how to help Larry. She admitted that Larry was very difficult to manage at home. In fact, she reported that she had given up trying to teach Larry how to behave. He was very rough with his siblings, bruising them and pulling their hair (his grandmother reported that his siblings had bald spots). She mentioned that Larry had almost set the house on fire while rewiring the toaster for an "experiment." He also experimented with cats in the neighborhood, pulling out their hair. His grandmother said that she had questioned Larry about the cats, but did not receive clear information about why he was harming them. His grandmother said, "I feel like I need to sleep with one eye open with Larry. I never know what he will do next and I don't think he cares for the feelings of others."

At his interview, Larry seemed somewhat detached and uncaring. He showed no emotion and never reported feelings of caring of others. Larry stated that he cut the girl's pigtail to test how sharp his scissors were. When asked about his friendships at school Larry replied, "They all know that I am the toughest kid in this school and I rule." Larry said he liked to rule others in his gang in the neighborhood, which he created. Larry said he created the "Rule Gang to be like the guys who have gangs in L.A. (Los Angeles)." When asked about his experiment with the toaster, Larry stated that he wanted to see if he could create fire. He reported that he and members of his school gang often met after school to try to start fires in the woods nearby the school. Larry admitted that he liked hurting cats. As far as his brothers and sisters, Larry said that he hurt them and did not really care about it.

The school counselor was alarmed at Larry's lack of feeling for other children and small animals. Larry did not feel he had to follow rules. He did not show empathy for others and appeared callous and unemotional. Larry did not appear to be forming close, loving relationships with any adults or children in his life. The counselor called a nearby children's mental health center with an inpatient unit. The counselor arranged an intake meeting with Larry and his grandmother. The school social worker arranged for a taxi to transport Larry and his grandmother to the mental health center.

At the intake session at the inpatient center, Larry admitted to killing a small cat to see what this felt like. He admitted to stealing money from his grandmother's wallet. Larry showed no remorse for harming others and stealing. He admitted to setting fires. He said he had rewired the toaster at home to turn it into a fire machine, because he wanted to try setting the house on fire. Larry admitted to setting many small fires in the woods and in his neighborhood.

Larry's grandmother cried during most of the interview. She said that, "I can't handle Larry, and his little sisters are so afraid of him. He hurts them every week and they have bruises and bald spots." Larry did not have any relatives who were willing for him to live with them. They had known of his aggressive and harmful behaviors and felt that he would harm others in their family. His mother could not be located. Larry's grandmother reported she did not want custody of Larry anymore and repeated that our family "can't handle him."

Larry was remanded to custody of the state and referred for an inpatient hospital stay. During this stay he participated in intensive therapy, group counseling, and was followed by a psychiatrist. His placement was at a juvenile center with other boys who had conduct problems. Treatment in this setting involved a great deal of supervision and structure. Children received rewards and privileges for appropriate behavior. They participated in daily group counseling and had their own individual counseling sessions. They were followed by a child psychiatrist. After completing his inpatient stay, he was going to be discharged to a therapeutic group home.

Summary

This chapter presented a brief overview of conduct problems in children. Behaviors that are disruptive to a significant degree, exemplify a marked disregard for social rules, and are aggressive can indicate serous conduct problems. For young children, parent interventions aimed at improving child social behavior and reducing negative behaviors (e.g., impulsivity, aggressiveness, and rule-breaking) may have an impact and reduce the chance that serious behavior problems will persist. Child training is important in order for children to learn social problem-solving skills and receive training to improve emotion regulation and friendship skills. Children need to learn to curb aggressive and hostile reactions. School-based training for teachers can be a critical component of an intervention program. There are many interventions, and those interventions that were presented in this chapter offer a brief glimpse of some of these effective interventions. Interested readers are encouraged to receive additional training and practice under supervision of experts in the field to gain experience in the treatment of conduct problems. Reduction in conduct problems can improve functioning of children, reduce school failure, and address patterns of aggression and rule-breaking behaviors that involve significant problems in social settings.

Exercises/Review Questions

1. What are key questions for assessment of conduct problems in children?
2. Is a genetic or environmental explanation more appropriate (or perhaps neither one) for the development of CD in children?
3. What is a hostile attribution bias? How could this be problematic in young children's peer interactions?
4. Search the internet for information about the Incredible Years Program. If you were running a community mental health center, would training in this program be beneficial for counselors in your program? Please provide details related to your opinion about this program.
5. What types of interventions would you focus on, if you were asked to develop a teacher training program for children with conduct problems? Please use the internet to search for ideas in addition to utilizing information presented in this chapter.

Key Concepts

Oppositional defiant disorder
Conduct disorder
Prosocial behaviors
Callous and unemotional traits
Problem-solving approach to working with children with conduct disorders
Modeling appropriate behaviors
Shaping appropriate behaviors
Hostile attributions toward others' behaviors
Fast Track Intervention
Positive time with children
Incredible Years Program
Turning to Kids Program

References

American Psychiatric Association. (2013). *Diagnostic and statistical manual of mental disorders* (5th ed.). Washington, DC: Author.

Andrade, B. F., & Tannock, R. (2012). The direct effects of inattention and hyperactivity/impulsivity on peer problems and mediating roles of prosocial and conduct problem behaviors in a community sample of children. *Journal of Attention Disorders, 17*(8), 670–680. doi:10.1177/1087054712437580.

Blair, R. J. R., Leibenluft, E., & Pine, D. S. (2014). Conduct disorder and callous–Unemotional traits in youth. *New England Journal of Medicine, 371*(23), 2207–2216.

Conduct Problems Prevention Research Group. (2011). The effects of the fast track preventive intervention on the development of conduct disorder across childhood. *Child Development, 82*(1), 331–345.

Dodge, K. A. (1980). Social cognition and children's aggressive behavior. *Child Development, 51*, 162–170.

Duncombe, M. E., Havighurst, S. S., Holland, K. A., & Frankling, E. J. (2012). Psychometric evaluation of a brief parent- and teacher-rated screen for children at risk of conduct disorder. *Australian Journal of Educational and Developmental Psychology, 12*, 1–11.

Eisenberg, N., Sadovsky, A., Spinrad, T. L., Fabes, R. A., Losoya, S., Valiente, C., … Shepard, S. A. (2005). The relations of problem behaviour status to children's negative emotionality, effortful control, and impulsivity: Concurrent relations and prediction of change. *Developmental Psychology, 41*, 193–211.

Frick, P. J., Ray, J. V., Thornton, L. C., & Kahn, R. E. (2013). Can callous-unemotional traits enhance the understanding, diagnosis, and treatment of serious conduct problems in children and adolescents? A comprehensive review. *Psychological Bulletin, 140*(1), 1–57. doi:10.1037/a0033076.

Furlong, M., McGilloway, S., Bywater, T., Hutchings, J., Smith, S. M., & Donnelly, M. (2013). Cochrane review: Behavioural and cognitive-behavioural group-based parenting programmes for early-onset conduct problems in children aged 3 to 12 years. *Evidence-Based Child Health: A Cochrane Review Journal, 8*(2), 318–692.

Havighurst, S. S., Duncombe, M., Frankling, E., Holland, K., Kehoe, C., & Stargatt, R. (2015). An emotion-focused early intervention for children with emerging conduct problems. *Journal of Abnormal Child Psychology, 43*(4), 749–760. doi:10.1007/s10802-014-9944-z.

Hawes, D. J., Price, M. J., & Dadds, M. R. (2014). Callous-unemotional traits and the treatment of conduct problems in childhood and adolescence: A comprehensive review. *Clinical Child and Family Psychology Review, 17*(3), 248–267. doi:10.1007/s10567-014-0167-1.

Herpertz, S. C., Mueller, B., Qunaibi, M., Lichterfeld, C., Konrad, K., & Herpertz-Dahlmann, B. (2005). Response to emotional stimuli in boys with conduct disorder. *American Journal of Psychiatry, 162*(6), 1100–1107.

Hutchings, J., Bywater, T., Daley, D., Gardner, F., Whitaker, C., Jones, K., … Edwards, R. T. (2007). Parenting intervention in Sure Start services for children at risk of developing conduct disorder: Pragmatic randomised controlled trial. *BMJ Online First, 334*(7595), e1–e7. doi:10.1136/bmj.39126.602799.55.

Kazdin, A. E. (1997). Practitioner review: Psychosocial treatments for conduct disorder in children. *Journal of Clinical Psychology and Psychiatry, 38*(2), 161–178.

Kim-Cohen, J., Arseneault, L., Caspi, A., Tomás, M. P., Taylor, A., & Moffitt, T. E. (2005). Validity of DSM-IV conduct disorder in 4 ½–5-year-old children: A longitudinal epidemiological study. *American Journal of Psychiatry, 162*(6), 1108–1117.

Maughan, B., & Rutter, M. (2001). Antisocial children grown up. In J. Hill & B. Maughan (Eds.), *Conduct disorders in childhood and adolescence* (pp. 507–552). Cambridge, England: Cambridge University Press.

Okado, Y., & Bierman, K. L. (2015). Differential risk for late adolescent conduct problems and mood dysregulation among children with early externalizing behavior problems. *Journal of Abnormal Child Psychology, 43*(4), 735–747.

Olson, S. L., Lopez-Duran, N., Lunkenheimer, E. S., Chang, H., & Sameroff, A. J. (2011). Individual differences in the development of early peer aggression: Integrating contributions of self-regulation, theory of mind, and parenting. *Development and Psychopathology, 23*, 253–266.

Patterson, G. R. (1982). *Coercive family process.* Eugene, OR: Castalia Press.

Patterson, G. R., & Stouthamer-Loeber, M. (1984). The correlation of family management practices and delinquency. *Child Development, 55*(4), 1299–1307.

Posthumus, J. A., Raaijmakers, M. A., Maassen, G. H., Van Engeland, H., & Matthys, W. (2012). Sustained effects of Incredible Years as a preventive intervention in preschool children with conduct problems. *Journal of Abnormal Child Psychology, 40*(4), 487–500.

Powell, N. P., Boxmeyer, C. L., Baden, R., Stromeyer, S., Minney, J. A., Mushtaq, A., & Lochman, J. E. (2011). Assessing and treating aggression and conduct problems in schools: Implications from the Coping Power program. *Psychology in the Schools, 48*(3), 233–242. doi: 10.1002/pits.20549.

Rouquette, A., Côté, S. M., Pryor, L. E., Carbonneau, R., Vitaro, F., & Tremblay, R. E. (2014). Cohort profile: The Quebec longitudinal study of kindergarten children (QLSKC). *International Journal of Epidemiology, 43*(1), 23–33. doi:10.1093/ije/dys177.

Silberg, J. L., Maes, H., & Eaves, L. J. (2012). Unraveling the effect of genes and environment in the transmission of parental antisocial behavior to children's conduct disturbance, depression and hyperactivity. *Journal of Child Psychology and Psychiatry, 53*(6), 668–677.

Tolan, P. H., Dodge, K., & Rutter, M. (2013). Tracking the multiple pathways of parent and family influence on disruptive behavior disorders. In P. H. Tolan & B. L. Leventhal (Eds.), *Disruptive behavior disorders, advances in developmental psychopathology: Brain research foundation symposium series* (pp. 161–192). New York, NY: Springer. doi:10.1007/978-1-4614-7557-6_7.

Webster-Stratton, C., & Reid, M. J. (2010). The Incredible Years parents, teachers, and children training services. In J. R. Weisz & A. E. Kazdin (Eds.), *Evidence-based psychotherapies for children and adolescents* (2nd ed., pp. 194–201). New York, NY: Guilford.

Webster-Stratton, C., Reid, M. J., & Hammond, M. (2004). Treating children with early conduct problems: Intervention outcomes for parent-, child- and teacher training. *Journal of Clinical Child and Adolescent Psychology, 33*, 221–239.

Wu, T., Howells, N., Burger, J., Lopez, P., Lundeen, R., & Sikkenga, A. V. (2015). Conduct disorder. In G. M. Kapalka (Ed.), *Treating disruptive disorders: A guide to psychological, pharmacological, and combined therapies* (pp. 120–143). New York, NY: Routledge.

Chapter 10
Attention-Deficit/Hyperactivity Disorder

Diagnosis

Children who have Attention-Deficit/Hyperactivity Disorder (ADHD) may have difficulty with sustaining their attention to important tasks as well as with controlling their impulsive and overactive behaviors. Specifically, children with ADHD may "… have difficulties with self-regulation, attention, working memory, cognitive flexibility, behavioral inhibition, and ability to sustain attention" (p. 551, Tamm, Nakonezny, & Hughes, 2014). Inability to control emotional reactions and regulate attention and concentration may be particularly difficult symptoms in school settings (Tamm et al., 2014). Children with ADHD may have a pattern of impulsivity and acting before they think, which are hallmark diagnostic features.

In the *Diagnostic and Statistical Manual of Mental Disorders* (American Psychiatric Association, 2013), ADHD is defined as, "A persistent pattern of inattention or hyperactivity-impulsivity that interferes with functioning or development." (p. 59). This is a diagnosis that is arrived upon after ruling out or making sure that the child does not have other types of problems, most notably conduct problems. Before concluding that one's diagnostic impression is ADHD the clinician also must be sure that the child has the cognitive and verbal abilities to understand how to complete tasks and to understand directions. The child needs to have displayed several of the symptoms of the disorder prior to 12 years of age. Furthermore, symptoms must be present across settings in the child's life, which are chiefly the home and school settings.

There are two main categories of symptoms to review before providing a diagnosis. These two categories are inattention and hyperactiveness as well as impulsive behaviors (American Psychiatric Association, 2013). In terms of the "inattention" category here are some common symptoms: failing to give attention to details, losing things, careless mistakes, and easily distracted by extraneous (not relevant) stimuli. These symptoms need to have been present for 6 or more months (American Psychiatric Association, 2013). A child with significant attention problems may be

© Springer International Publishing Switzerland 2016
L. Nabors, *Medical and Mental Health During Childhood*, Springer
Series on Child and Family Studies, DOI 10.1007/978-3-319-31117-3_10

likely to be "off-task" in the classroom and therefore not completing assignments. This child also might forget to write down or complete class assignments or forget to do his or her daily chores. The second category is hyperactivity-impulsivity. Examples of symptoms in this category include: fidgets or squirms, runs and/or climbs in situations where it is not appropriate to do so, blurts out answers, talks incessantly, and has difficulty waiting his or her turn. The diagnosis of ADHD may be either: a predominantly inattentive presentation, a predominantly hyperactive/impulsive presentation, or a combined presentation in which symptoms in both of the categories are present. The clinician also specifies a severity level for the child's symptoms—mild, moderate, or severe.

There are age differences in the presentation of symptoms. Although difficulties with poor planning skills and inattention as well as restlessness can persist into the adolescent years, these symptoms are most "noticeable" during childhood (American Psychiatric Association, 2013). In preschool, the main symptom children display is hyperactivity. It is considered somewhat difficult to provide or "make" the diagnosis of ADHD before 4 years of age.

Prevalence of Attention-Deficit Hyperactivity Disorder in Children

Rates of ADHD may vary across studies (Pliszka & the AACAP Working Group, 2007). For instance, Larson, Russ, Kahn, and Halfon (2011) proposed that rates of ADHD in children were about 8 % based on parent report. A majority of children diagnosed with ADHD (from 60 to 85 %) will continue to meet criteria for the disorder in adolescence (Pliszka & the AACAP Working Group, 2007). Rates for ADHD in young adulthood may vary between 2 and 8 %. Even though some persons may no longer meet the full criteria for this disorder in adulthood, they may continue to experience symptoms that interfere with their daily functioning. Boys are more likely to be diagnosed with ADHD compared to girls. In fact, the male to female ratio is 2:1 (American Psychiatric Association, 2013). Females, if diagnosed, are more likely to be diagnosed with symptoms of inattention.

Genetic and Environmental Influences. ADHD has genetic precursors and has been correlated with several different genes. Like many mental health conditions, ADHD can "run in families." In neuroimaging studies of children with ADHD, who have not been treated with medication, scans have revealed that there was reduced cortical white and gray matter. There also were differences for children who had received medication, but differences were not as pronounced (not as great; Pliszka & the AACAP Group, 2007). Although it is always difficult to separate environmental from genetic influences, it may be that children residing in families experiencing adversity, such as residing in low-income, inner city environments where there is violence and family conflict, may have children with increased vulnerability to ADHD symptomatology (Biederman, Faraone, & Monuteaux, 2002). The exact cause for this disorder has yet to be determined. Interactions between genetic and environmental factors probably are related to the development of this disorder.

Impacts on Children and Parents

ADHD can co-occur with several other health and mental health problems. For example, children with ADHD can have sleep problems. They have higher rates of being diagnosed with epilepsy and may exhibit other types of neurological symptoms (American Psychiatric Association, 2013). Children with ADHD may be more likely to have different types of learning disabilities and other types of psychiatric problems than children without this condition (Larson et al., 2011). Larson et al. found that learning disabilities were very common in children with ADHD followed by conduct problems. They also discovered that children with ADHD may be more likely to repeat a grade in school and have school-related problems compared to children who are developing typically. Watson, Richels, Michalek, and Raymer (2015) conducted a very comprehensive review of the treatment literature and found that information is lacking about best practices for treating children with ADHD who have learning disorders. Children with ADHD may experience depression and anxiety at higher rates than children without this problem; however, conduct problems are likely to be more common than internalizing problems, like anxiety and depression. Larson et al. reported that children with ADHD were likely to use health and mental health services at higher rates than children with other types of mental health problems. Rates of comorbid or co-occurring problems in children who have ADHD may be influenced by family socioeconomic status. Larson et al. reported that children from very low-income families were more likely to have other types of learning and mental health problems than children residing in families with higher income levels. Larson et al. concluded that when working with children who have ADHD it is imperative to screen for other mental health and health problems to provide them with the most comprehensive treatment possible.

Children with the combined presentation of ADHD, with both inattentive and hyperactive-impulsive symptoms, may have comorbid, or co-occurring "acting out" behavior problems. In the practice parameters document developed by Pliszka and the American Academy of Child and Adolescent Psychiatry Work Group on Quality Issues (2007), it was noted that, "...54–84 % of children and adolescents with ADHD may meet criteria for oppositional defiant disorder (ODD); a significant portion of these patients will develop conduct disorder." (p. 896). The experts for the AACAP working group reported that children with ADHD may have deficits in executive functions, which are neurological and cognitive skills that allow a child to solve a problem to organize and attain a future goal. The problems with executive functions can mean deficits in inhibiting responses, paying attention to important or key tasks, organizing materials, memory, and planning.

Having a child with ADHD can have a significant impact on parental stress and well-being (Theule, Wiener, Tannock, & Jenkins, 2013). Parents may benefit from training to help their child learn to manage impulsive behaviors and reduce negative behaviors. Bennett, Barlow, Huband, Smailagic, and Roloff (2013) indicated that parents benefitted from attending parent training programs. Parents of children with ADHD may benefit from parent training in that it will give them ideas for providing structure for their child, in terms of consistent teaching techniques to help their child learn limits for impulsive and/or negative behaviors. Parents could experience reductions in anxiety, anger, guilt, and stress after attending training programs. These gains might be short-term; therefore, Bennett et al. recommended long-term support for parents.

Theule, Wiener, Rogers, and Marton (2013) reported that parents may benefit from the support they receive for their own self-care and stress relief that they find when attending parenting groups. Parenting groups need to be multifaceted, providing education about ADHD, ideas for problem-solving at home and at school, and education about support and stress relief for parents. If the child is exhibiting significant oppositional and defiant behaviors or if one of the child's parents had ADHD, then parental support may be critical to positive family and child functioning.

Assessment

Pliszka and the AACAP Group (2007; http://www.jaacap.com/article/S089-0-8567(09)62182-1/pdf; downloaded July 7, 2015) recommended that clinicians review symptoms in the DSM when making diagnoses. The symptoms must cause significant impairment in several settings or contexts of the child's life. These experts recommended asking parents about symptoms related to acting out problems, especially oppositional behaviors and conduct problems. Clinicians need to ask questions to determine child intellectual functioning as well as screen for learning problems. Family history of ADHD and history of ADHD for parents also need to be assessed. Interviewing the child will provide critical information about his or her view of possible symptoms.

Moreover, experts suggest that parents and teachers complete rating scales to document symptoms of ADHD. It is noteworthy that there are many good scales for assessment of ADHD. The Vanderbilt ADHD Diagnostic Parent and Teacher Scales (Wolraich, Lambert, Baumgaertel, et al., 2003; Wolraich, Lambert, Doffing, et al., 2003) are two scales used by professionals. The Bright Futures Program posted a copy of the Vanderbilt Teacher Rating Scale (https://brightfutures.org/mentalhealth/pdf/professionals/bridges/adhd.pdf). A copy of the Vanderbilt Parent Rating Scale is available at this website: http://www.ncfahp.org/Data/Sites/1/media/images/pdf/CHIP-Vanderbilt-parent.pdf. The scales and directions for using and scoring them are also available at http://www.nichq.org/childrens-health/adhd/resources/vanderbilt-assessment-scales, a website developed by the NICHQ, which is the National

Institute for Children's Health Quality [http://www.nichq.org/about/organization; websites in this paragraphs were accessed on July 8, 2015].

These two scales are available free of charge and are well-established surveys. Parents and teachers complete these scales by rating their perceptions of symptoms of ADHD and co-occurring problems. When using the aforementioned scales, clinicians should remember that parent and teacher agreement on symptoms of ADHD may be low (e.g., Wolraich et al., 2004). This may occur because teachers and parents focus on different behaviors. It may be that behaviors are more prevalent or noticeable at school, because symptoms of ADHD may be more noticeable in group settings. If this is the case, then teacher ratings could appear more "severe" than parent ratings. On the other hand, it may be that teachers are able to provide structure or have experience with ADHD and these things could influence their ratings, making their ratings more positive than those provided by parents. There may be other reasons as well, but because there can be differences across settings and informants, it is important to supplement data from surveys with data from interviews and observations.

Disease Management

There are many ideas for management of ADHD to promote child functioning. The ideas presented in this section of the chapter are based on the author's clinical experiences working with parents of children with ADHD to improve their behaviors at home and at school. In terms of at home, children with ADHD may have difficulty following instructions. Parents may need to turn off the television and avoid extraneous noise and distractions when providing instructions to their child. For some children it may be advisable to write down instructions or have a chart on the refrigerator with chores or important "to do" tasks. Whenever possible, encourage parents to use praise and small, immediate rewards to encourage positive behaviors. A child with ADHD often responds better to immediate feedback and positive information about what he or she is doing. This type of feedback can help all children, but structure, routine, and immediate feedback may be especially helpful for a child who has ADHD.

In terms of discipline, response cost and time-out are recommended. A response cost occurs with the child who behaves in a negative way and experiences a loss of a privilege. Parents should not take away a privilege for too long or to take too many privileges away, because a child can feel hopeless and then "give up" on working toward exhibiting more positive behaviors. Children with ADHD may make excuses for their behavior. Being matter of fact and talking about what is expected of the child during calm periods may help a parent to teach a child. The parent could then ignore excuses and mention that he or she has explained positive behaviors and consequences for negative behaviors. This may reduce arguing that can result in a negative exchange between parent and child. Another discipline technique is a time-out, where a child sits in a chair for 1 min for each year of age. A time-out period provides a child with a chance to calm down and understand that some behaviors are not acceptable. A child should not to be able to entertain him- or herself in time-out. The child should lack stimulation in the time-out chair or area. If the child argues in time-out, the parent should not argue back, because a child should be "bored" during the time-out period. Parents should not overuse time-outs and should select specific behaviors for which there is a time-out. Following through consistently is recommended. The discipline techniques described in this paragraph work well for all children. They may be especially helpful for children who experience hyperactivity.

Children with ADHD may thrive on "structure." It typically is important to instruct the parent to give clear instructions and act the same way in terms of following through on instructions and consequences for behavior. Lists of what to do after school can be helpful. For example, a simple list might read, "(1) Snack, (2) Homework, and (3) Play." When the child comes inside from play, it is time to wash hands, set the table, and sit quietly until dinner is served. Reviewing lists with the child in his or her own words can be helpful. Some children may need time limits for completion of tasks. These limits can be set using a timer, keeping track on a clock visible to the child, or using the alarm on a cellular telephone. If the child is overwhelmed in a certain environment, reducing distractions may assist the child in focusing on tasks that need to be completed. If a task is too large or directions are too long, then breaking a task or information into manageable "chunks" can help a child succeed in completing a task, or following instructions.

Children with ADHD can lose things. Therefore, instruct parents to develop a homework station and routine and/or a checklist for completing homework. The child should place finished homework in a "finished" folder in his or her backpack. Backpacks should be kept in a chair by the door. This routine should be followed every night and the child should be reminded to check his or her backpack to ensure completed homework is in the right place. In the majority of cases, it is recommended that parents tell the child's teacher about the child's diagnosis and develop a Section 504 Plan to record interventions that will help the child at school. If problem behaviors occur regularly, then parents should ask teachers to send home a note each night. Parents should encourage and reward appropriate classroom behaviors as well as well-done homework.

Parents can request a list of homework assignments with due dates and ask for calendars with due dates. If a child is having difficulty recalling the rules at school, the parent can ask the teacher about school rules and set up a similar structure at home. Sometimes children with ADHD benefit from being seated close to the teacher, so that the teacher can encourage paying attention and completion of work. Working on group tasks in a group where there is a child who can act as a role model can also be helpful. The child may need a reward chart for working well with others at school. A special signal (thumbs up sign) or verbal reminder (e.g., let's focus now) from the teacher can be a reminder for the child, signaling to the child that he or she needs to be "on task" completing the assignment at hand.

Linking parents to supports is another important goal. One source of information and support is the website for CHADD (http://www.chadd.org/; accessed on July 8, 2015), Children and Adults with Attention-Deficit/Hyperactivity Disorder, a national-level organization providing education, advocacy, and support for adults and children with ADHD. The aforementioned website has guidance for parents and caregivers on many different subjects, including management of child ADHD symptoms at home and at school. Another resource for parents is the ADD Warehouse (http://www.addwarehouse.com/shopsite_sc/store/html/index.html; accessed on July 8, 2015), where parents can purchase books, planners, and other tools. Both of the aforementioned resources are tools for health professionals as well, with helpful resources to guide them in their work with children and their families.

A useful book for working with the children is, "Putting on the Brakes: Understanding and Taking Control of your ADD or ADHD: Second Edition," by Quinn and Stern (2008). This book is for children aged 9 and older, but many of the explanations can be used with children as young as seven. The book has a companion activity book entitled, "Putting on the Brakes Activity Book for Kids with ADD or ADHD" (Quinn & Stern, 2009). This book has activities for children that explain their ADHD and offers strategies for coping with ADHD. A book that can help children to understand how their medication works and the importance of taking their medication is entitled, "Otto Learns about his Medicine: A Story about Medication for Children with ADHD, Third Edition" (Galvin, 2001). For young elementary school-age youth and preschool children other resources for explaining symptoms that will help alleviate misunderstanding are available. One book that might be useful in teaching children about their symptoms is entitled, "Eukee the Jumpy Jumpy Elephant," by Corman and Trevino (2009). Another book is, "Shelley the Hyperactive Turtle" by Deborah Moss (2006). This book explains how Shelley, a small turtle, is different from many other young turtles because he is very active and has trouble remaining quiet. Shelley is described as smart and handsome, and in very positive terms.

Children with ADHD may suffer from low self-esteem. Thus, it is advisable for parents to find things their child does well, is keenly interested in and excels at, so that their child can build a sense of accomplishment and feelings of self-worth. Reminding children with ADHD about their strengths and how they are special will help in combatting feelings of low self-worth.

Medications

Medications may be successful in the treatment of the behavioral symptoms, especially negative behaviors, associated with ADHD (Antshel, 2015). Stimulant medications are commonly used treatments for children with ADHD. Methylphenidates are often prescribed and names for these medications include Concerta, Focalin, and Ritalin (Dulcan & AACAP Workgroup on Quality Issues, 1997). Amphetamines may be used to treat symptoms of ADHD. Examples of this class of drug are Adderall or Vyvanse. When pediatricians and psychiatrists begin giving a medication, they often start with a lower dose, frequently check child progress, and then move to a higher dose. This careful monitoring and dose adjustment is common. At office visits, pediatricians and psychiatrists also will monitor child weight and height. There are other medications that are used and medication management can be very complex (a detailed review is beyond the scope of this chapter). It is noteworthy, that there is less information on the use of medications with very young children (e.g., preschoolers).

Both long-acting and short-acting forms of the medication are effective (Dulcan & AACAP Workgroup on Quality Issues, 1997; Pliszka & the AACAP Working Group, 2007). For some children the long-acting medications are easier to take because they are administered one time each day. However, when the longer acting medication is finished, some children can have a rebound effect where they become active or moody. In these cases, the child might need a short-acting medicine to help them in the evening, such as when they are completing their homework. The medications are considered relatively mild, in terms of side effects. They can negatively influence child appetite and sleep. If the child is not eating well and needs to "catch up" on eating and "growing," then medication holidays may be appropriate. Medication holidays occur when the child does not take the medication over the summer or holiday breaks from school. These breaks can allow children who have a loss of appetite to catch up (in terms of eating and growing). Other side effects can be headaches, mood changes (i.e., mood swings), or motor ticks (Cortese et al., 2013). Due to difficulty with psychosocial functioning, medications should probably be used along with behavioral and psychosocial interventions to fully treat symptoms associated with ADHD (Antshel, 2015; MTA Cooperative Group, 1999).

Psychosocial and Emotional Functioning

Problems in social, interpersonal, and family interactions have been discovered for children with ADHD (Abikoff et al., 2004; Antshel, 2015). Problems with social interactions can impede social development and cause long-term problems for children. Research shows that ADHD has a negative impact on children's quality of life (Danckaerts et al., 2010). Quality of life is a complex construct or idea, associated with a child's well-being, which is derived from his or her perceptions of his or her social, academic, and family functioning. In a comprehensive review, Danckaerts et al. (2010) found that some children with ADHD see their quality of life as impaired compared to children without this disorder. Although children may have a positive view of their lives, it is likely that their parents have a negative view of the impact of their ADHD and feel that symptoms of ADHD are negatively impacting their children's lives.

Children with ADHD have difficulty controlling impulsive behaviors and this can be very difficult in social situations. They may blurt out answers, not follow instructions, not complete tasks, and have difficulty transitioning when engaged in activity, making it difficult for them to "get along" and fit in during different social experiences, such as school, neighborhood activities with peers, or sports events. As mentioned, children with ADHD often have other psychological problems and learning problems, which also adds stress and may further disrupt social and academic functioning (American Psychiatric Association, 2013; Pliszka & the AACAP Working Group, 2007). Because ADHD has a profound impact on a child's behavioral functioning and his or her abilities to get along with others, interventions to improve social functioning, along with medication management, are very important for children with ADHD (Barkley, 2014). Also, interventions to improve child school functioning, planning, and organization can have a positive impact on child functioning. These types of interventions are discussed to in the next section of this chapter.

Interventions for Children with ADHD

Perhaps the most comprehensive study of the treatment of ADHD is the MTA Study (MTA is the abbreviation for the NIMH Collaborative Multisite Multimodal Treatment Study of Children with Attention-Deficit/Hyperactivity Disorder), where a national review of ADHD treatments was conducted (e.g., MTA Cooperative Group, 1999). There were four groups for this study, representing children treated with methylphenidate alone, psychosocial treatment alone, a combination of medication management and psychosocial treatment, and community treatment. For medication management, doses were carefully modified by physicians based on information from parent and teacher reports. The psychosocial treatment was very thorough. Children participated in a summer camp to learn critical strategies for managing their ADHD. Parents participated in parent groups, with intensive coaching available above and beyond the management training from the groups. Teachers participated in consultation sessions where they learned strategies for helping children with ADHD. Classroom support for children was available. Study results indicated that children in all four treatment groups showed declines in symptoms related to ADHD after 14 months in treatment. The two groups receiving medication management showed better outcomes than those in the psychosocial treatment alone or the community treatment groups (MTA Cooperative Group, 1999).

Interestingly, the children in the community treatment group often received medications, but the use of medications were not monitored in the same stringent manner as those in the two medication groups (medication and medication plus psychosocial treatment; MTA Cooperative Group, 1999). The community group had a lower degree of follow-up in terms of checking medication management. It was concluded that these children may have been treated with lower doses of medications that were therefore not as effective as could have been possible. Approximately 25 % of the children in the psychosocial treatment group also needed some medication management at some point during the course of their care. The researchers concluded that medication management may be a necessary factor for successful management of ADHD symptoms, especially negative behaviors related to impulse control.

After the 14-month study had ended, the treatment groups were no longer followed in the same way. The medication management group and the combined group (with psychosocial treatment and medication management) were "handed off to community physicians" (p. 760) for treatment as usual (MTA Cooperative Group, 2004a). When treatment had ended and regular community supports were initiated, medication doses tended to decrease and the supports associated with stringent medication management were no longer in place. For many participants medication use declined. Results of a follow-up assessment at 24 months showed that some of the initial benefits related to the stringent medication management appeared to be declining once this intensive management was removed (MTA Cooperative Group, 2004a). Although treatment had ended, children who participated in the two medication groups (medication management and medication plus psychosocial treatment) were still exhibiting gains in positive functioning. Children in the combined group (medication plus psychosocial treatment) exhibited fewer oppositional defiant behaviors, relatively better social skills, and their parents were showing advantages in using discipline. The authors of the follow-up study concluded that these findings provided some support for the notion that psychosocial treatment was a useful adjunctive treatment when medication management was used (MTA Cooperative Group, 2004a). They reported that a combination treatment could result in lower use of medications for ADHD. This could attenuate the negative side effects from using higher doses of stimulant medications (e.g., motor ticks). Despite these positive findings, a major finding was that the positive impact of intensive treatment was beginning to decrease, even though gains were still evident.

The positive outcomes were not maintained at a 6–8 year follow-up of the MTA groups (Molina et al., 2009). The MTA groups were not improved over the normative comparison group (that did not receive treatment) at long-term follow-up. The use of medication had significantly declined in MTA groups. After 6–8 years, the best predictor of how the children were functioning was the severity of their symptoms. Specifically, children with more severe symptoms and both inattentive and hyperactive/impulse behaviors had a worse prognosis than other children. The gains for the children in the MTA study were thought to last at the 36-month assessment period. The researchers conducting the 6–8 year follow-up did note that children residing in low-income families were likely to be lost to follow-up assessments. Study results may have overestimated children's positive functioning. The researchers suggested that continued treatment may be needed, especially for children with more severe symptoms, as they reach adolescence. The researchers conducting the follow-up study called for research on factors supporting adolescents through the adult years and supporting families in the long-term as their child with ADHD matures and faces new challenges (Molina et al., 2009).

Abikoff et al. (2004) reviewed information on treatment of social problems in children with ADHD. In their review of relevant literature, they found that treatment with stimulant medications, such as methylphenidate, can reduce negative social behaviors. They reported that psychosocial treatment, such as social skills training, has been touted as a potential intervention to improve social development. Abikoff et al. mentioned that there is limited support for the effectiveness of social skills training and other types of training, when children are not medicated to help them improve their attention and concentration.

Abikoff et al. (2004) conducted a study to determine what would occur if two types of psychosocial treatments were added to medication treatment. The boys and girls who participated in this study were between 8 and 11 years of age. Children were randomly assigned to groups to receive methylphenidate alone, methylphenidate plus PATHKO social skills training, and methylphenidate plus organizational skills training. There also was a wait-list control group. A goal for this study was to compare teaching of organizational skills to a behaviorally based, social skills intervention, and determine the impact of the two types of training on social skills. As mentioned, children did not receive treatment in the wait-list control group, but this only occurred for a small part of the study. The children in the wait-list control group needed to receive some type of treatment after a few months, in order to help them. Ensuring that children in wait-list control groups receive needed treatments is part of the ethical conduct of a research study.

PATHKO stood for Parents and Teachers Helping Kids Organize (Abikoff et al., 2004). The PATHKO treatment was considered multimodal in that it addressed strategies for improving children's organizational skills, social skills, as well as academic assistance, and it included psychotherapy for children with ADHD. Parents participated in weekly training in the first year of the study and they attended monthly parent training sessions during the second year of the study. Teachers completed report cards to provide information to parents about the children's progress at school, and the children's parents rewarded progress at school after review of positive information about behavior on the report cards. Social skills training for the children involved learning ways to get along with peers, training in conversational skills, and problem-solving with plans for trouble-shooting problem situations and interactions.

In contrast, the organizational skills training involved learning to organize classroom work, turn in assignments, manage handouts, use calendars and planners, and utilize homework completion and backpack checklists (a checkllist to ensure all finished work was placed in the backpack; Abikoff et al., 2004). Moreover, children in the organizational skills training group learned how to plan their time to complete homework and long-term assignments. Parents learned how to supervise homework and reward children for positive behaviors.

Abikoff et al. (2004) found that children in the methylphenidate group, PATHKO plus methylphenidate group, and organizational skills training group plus methylphenidate group showed improvements in social skills. Both parents and teachers rated improved performance in social skills for children in the aforementioned groups. The important thing to consider for this study is that the PATHKO treatment and organizational skills treatment had high costs added, without significant gains for children, compared to the methylphenidate-alone group. That is, children receiving methylphenidate alone, without the additional treatments, improved to a similar degree as the children in the other groups. These authors believed this was due to the positive impact that methylphenidate has on reducing problem behaviors, which can result in negative social interactions. If negative behaviors decrease, the child may learn positive behaviors due to increased abilities to focus, without the need for intensive psychosocial intervention. One might have thought that the PATHKO training would have been more effective than the organizational skills training. This was not the case, perhaps because each intervention used similar techniques to assist children and parents. It is noteworthy that children in the organizational skills training group did show some gains in academic functioning. Improving organizational skills may improve school performance, and may be more cost-effective than some intensive interventions. Children in this study had above average intellectual functioning and this may have influenced study results. More research assessing the benefits of psychosocial treatments will provide knowledge about whether these types of treatments add benefit for children with ADHD who exhibit below-average intellectual functioning.

Although Abikoff et al. (2004) did not find added benefits to psychosocial treatment, the results of the MTA Study (2004b), a national-level study, indicated that behavioral therapy, along with teacher and parent training, can be advantageous when combined with medication. The MTA study is considered a gold standard, and the results of this study supported the implementation of multimodal therapy, with behavioral therapy and child, parent, and teacher training, and medication management as best practice in treatment of ADHD. On the other hand, psychosocial treatments may be less effective when children are not receiving stringent medication management to ensure they have a correct dose of medication. Pfiffner et al. (2014) conducted a study examining the influence of a comprehensive treatment (the Child Life and Attentive Skills Program; CLAS Program). This treatment program included child, parent, and teacher training using the CLAS program. Pfiffner et al. compared treatment with this program to treatment as usual for children with ADHD who had predominantly inattentive symptoms. Teacher ratings showed child gains in social functioning, organizational skills, and attention. Their results indicated that comprehensive training of children, parents, and teachers was superior to treatment as usual. Pfiffner et al. recommended psychosocial treatments for child, parent, and teacher as best practices in helping children cope with ADHD.

After conducting a review of many studies, Watson et al. (2015) proposed that multimodal interventions to support the child, parent, and teacher combined with medication management might be considered a current "best practice" in supporting children with ADHD and their parents. Watson et al. recommended training teachers, especially in cases where school functioning is at risk for children with ADHD. Behavioral interventions involve rewards for positive classroom behaviors and school–home notes to provide parents with information about school performance so that they may reinforce positive behaviors that were exhibited at school when they review the report card at home. More research is needed to determine what components of behavioral interventions are successful for children under different circumstances and with different types of comorbid conditions. Watson et al. (2015) pointed out that information is lacking about the optimal interventions for children with ADHD and different types of learning disabilities. Learning about interventions for children with learning problems will be a critical area for future research.

Another promising treatment for very young children who have symptoms of ADHD may be training to improve skills related to executive functioning. Tamm et al. (2014) noted that medication management, though positive, may not always alleviate problems related to executive functions, because children may continue to have difficulty with organizational and planning abilities. Tamm et al. described executive functions as allowing a child to organize information in memory, plan courses of action, and develop and evaluate appropriate courses of action from organizing information from the environment. In summary, executive function skills promote control and organization of cognitive (thinking) operations that allow one to organize information, plan, and act in one's environment. They observed that early intervention in the preschool years, when parents and children are at early stages of working with ADHD symptoms, may be an optimal time for interventions. These researchers recruited preschool children to participate in an intervention to improve executive functioning. Children participated in small groups where they participated in activities, such as completing puzzles and search games (where children find hidden objects in pictures), that promoted executive functioning. The interventionists, who lead the small groups, praised children's efforts at paying attention and praised their search strategies. The interventionists also used behavior management techniques that were appropriate for young children who had difficulty managing their attention and overactive behaviors. Parents participated in training sessions where they learned to implement games addressing search strategies, attention, and memory. At the end of the training sessions, parents and preschool teachers reported improvements in children's behaviors and improved attention. The intervention was practical and attendance in the parent groups was good. Tamm et al. concluded that the long-term outcomes of interventions to improve executive functioning in young children need to be investigated because "executive control processes appear to be central in the etiology (cause) of externalizing behavior disorders" (p. 557, Tamm et al., 2014). They proposed that effortful control of executive functions can be taught and can improve behavioral functioning, even for very young children.

Roles for Health Educators

Health educators can play a key role in educating teachers, parents, and children about the symptoms of ADHD as well as teaching about the differences between the inattentive and hyperactive "types" of this disorder. Parents and teachers may not know that inattentive symptoms are more common in girls. Parents and teachers need to learn about the importance of structure and improving executive functioning skills for many children with ADHD. Many may feel that medication management is not successful or that medications for ADHD are an attempt to "overmedicate" the child. In translating the literature for parents and teachers, health educators may help them realize that medication works to help the child focus and reduce impulsive behaviors. This education may help them to improve their perceptions of medication use, so that children can benefit from this treatment.

Health educators can also facilitate the child's school success and success in extracurricular activities by providing ideas for teachers and coaches. The ideal teacher and coach will provide structure and use routines. These adults will communicate clearly, repeating instructions as necessary. They will use lists and visual reminders of assignments or key things that the child needs to remember. They will help the child remember to take turns when engaging in conversations, listen to others, and let other children express opinions as well as take the lead during social activities. The health educator can refer the parent and child to local support groups, if they are available. The health educator can provide important referrals for tutoring and other parent supports, such referral to experts at local children's hospitals.

Case Study

Jessie was an elementary school-age girl with a younger sister, who was in pre-school. She and her parents lived nearby some of her family members. She had few friends, because she was likely to be perceived as "bossy" and taking over leadership of group activities. She is viewed, according to her parents, as having difficulty getting along in groups. Jessie has had difficulty in school since kindergarten. She is currently in the third grade and her teachers have been very concerned with her functioning. She has forgotten to complete her school work, talks in class, has difficulty following instructions and completing assignments in the classroom, and difficulty remaining seated during lecture and small group activities. She typically plays alone on the playground. Her classmates do not invite her to play games, because she has difficulty following the rules and keeping up with the pace of their playground activities.

Jessie's father reported that he had been diagnosed with "ADD" as a child. He had difficulty in school and often thought of himself as being "bad," because he could not focus on his work. Jessie's father completed high school; but, he dropped out of college after his freshman year, because he could not keep up with assignments. Currently, her father holds a job as a truck driver, which is well suited to him, because he likes to stay up at night and make his own schedule. He functions well under the structure of a deadline for getting a shipment delivered. Jessie's mother also had trouble paying attention in college, but was able to complete her bachelor's degree in Marketing. She currently works part-time from their home. Jessie gets along fairly well with her younger sister, but she has to be "large and in charge" of all that is happening. Her parents, similar to her teacher, have become frustrated with her lack of follow-through when they give her instructions and the difficulties she has with transitioning from one activity to another. Similar to her teacher, they noted that her pencil grip is awkward, and her handwriting seems behind for a child in her age range. Jessie often returns home feeling upset after playing with other children in the neighborhood, Her parents are worried that she is getting a reputation for not getting along well with other children.

Jessie is likely to "talk back" at home. She has difficulty with arguing if her parents ask her to do something. She always feels she is "right" and she makes excuses rather quickly for the mistakes she makes. Despite her tendencies to defend herself, her parents feel that Jessie is suffering from low self-esteem, and that she realizes that she is having a difficult time getting along at home and at school. When her school counselor talked with Jessie, she admitted, "I am not feeling so great about myself." Jessie's pediatrician noticed that over the years Jessie continued to experience difficulties with paying attention, completing tasks, impulsivity, and hyperactive behaviors. Her pediatrician asked Jessie's mother to sign a release of information so that she could speak with Jessie's school counselor and provide information to her teachers. Her pediatrician and the school counselor spoke by telephone. This allowed her pediatrician to learn that problems with impulsivity, attention, and overactivity were present in the school setting.

Her pediatrician asked Jessie's mother to complete the Vanderbilt Parent Rating Scale. The pediatrician also sent the Vanderbilt Teacher Rating Scale to Jessie's teacher. When the Vanderbilt Parent and Teacher Rating Scales were scored the total scores indicated that Jessie was experiencing significant problems with activity level, impulsivity, attention, and concentration both at home and at school. This was corroborated by interview information, both from Jessie's mother and school personnel. The pediatrician was very comfortable with the treatment of ADHD in children; it was a specialty area for her. A first step was providing the diagnosis to Jessie's parents, which the pediatrician did during a parent session. Her parents were accepting of the diagnosis. Jessie's pediatrician was thankful for their agreement, because in her experience, parents did not always agree with a diagnosis or recommendations for a medication trial, which was the recommendation for Jessie.

The pediatrician recommended Ritalin, beginning at a low dose. Jessie responded to being on the medication almost immediately, showing improvements in her classroom behavior. However, the medication, which was short-acting, was not helping at home. A small dose, given after she came home from school, was added after a period of time. Jessie's teacher reported improved attention. More homework assignments were completed. After beginning to use medication, few homework assignments were missing and all classroom assignments were completed. Jessie had fewer issues with, "talking out of turn and blurting out answers," according to her teacher. Jessie had been referred to a social skills group with her school counselor and she was responding well to the new information she learned in the group. Her behaviors with peers on the playground had vastly improved. Her teacher was using frequent reminders for Jessie to "stay on track" and complete her work. She was making sure Jessie wrote down her homework assignments in her planner. These behavioral "reminders" and "checks" were helping Jessie to complete her work.

Things at home, in terms of the arguing with parents, had not improved. Her parents were engaging in daily "battles" with Jessie to complete her chores and school work. Although she always completed her homework, usually just in the "nick of time," she was not completing her chores around the house. She was especially argumentative with her mother. Upon hearing of this issue, Jessie's pediatrician called the school counselor who agreed to have a few parent training sessions with Jessie's parents. The information shared in these sessions would help her parents establish a chore chart, with written expectations for her household chores. Her parents learned to use time-out in her room as a method for discipline when her arguing got "out of control." She would go to her room for 10 min and could return to be with the family, if her arguing ceased. The school counselor and Jessie's parents decided to try this technique after they gained insight that Jessie was responding to the negative attention she received from arguing. The school counselor also provided referrals to a local children's hospital, at the ADHD Children's clinic, for parenting groups for parents of children with ADHD. The school counselor and parents agreed to follow-up with another meeting in 2 weeks, to determine whether their behavior management plans were facilitating positive changes at home. Jessie's pediatrician was going to meet with Jessie and her parents every 3 months for medication management, in order to ensure that the medication was helpful and to check Jessie's height and weight.

Summary

In this chapter information about the diagnosis, management, and treatment of ADHD was reviewed. This disorder is heterogeneous in nature, with many different presentations and implications for children. Children with ADHD can present with a myriad of learning or psychological problems. Their parents may also have ADHD, as this disorder tends to run in families. When this occurs, it may be necessary to educate the parent about his or her own ADHD and provide referrals to a psychologist or psychiatrist for the parent. Children with ADHD may benefit from medication management, which will help reduce impulsive behaviors and help them focus, so that they can maximally benefit from behavioral interventions. Combined medication and psychosocial treatment may be the most effective treatment for a child with ADHD. Psychosocial treatments involve several components, such as use of structure, reinforcement, organizational training, etc. Children with ADHD thrive on structure and clear limit-setting, as do many children. Many children with ADHD benefit from homework routines to ensure that they have a "set" way of completing homework. Parent training may be needed to teach parents behavioral skills to help their child manage symptoms of ADHD. Symptoms of ADHD may seem to lessen in severity as children age, because they may be less active. For many children with ADHD, symptoms will remain in some form; so, learning how to manage their symptoms and cope better at school and at home can be a protective factor for years to come.

Exercises/Review Questions
1. If you were asked to educate teachers about helping children with ADHD what types of key topics would you address?
2. Conduct a web search and locate the Vanderbilt Teacher Rating Scale and the Vanderbilt Parent Rating Scale. Review each measure thoroughly. Next answer (a) and (b) below.

(a) What are your opinions of these measures?

(b) What types of interview questions would you use to uncover further information from teachers and parents, in addition to the information gained from using these measures?

3. What are executive functions?

4. What was the MTA study and what were the key findings from this study?

5. What types of computer games would you create to help children with ADHD learn planning and organizational skills?

6. If you were planning a social skills training session for a child with ADHD, what types of skills would you be reviewing? Please name at least two skills you would review and focus on how you would provide examples and clear instructions for a child with ADHD to attain each skill.

Key Concepts
Symptoms associated with ADHD
2 categories of symptoms for ADHD (inattentive and hyperactive-impulsive type)
ADHD, Combined Type
Vanderbilt Scales
Response cost
Structure for children with ADHD
Methylphenidate
Medication holiday
Multimodal Treatment Study (MTA Study)
PATHKO training
Executive functioning

References

Abikoff, H., Hechtman, L., Klein, R. G., Gallagher, R., Fleiss, K., Etcovitch, J. O. Y., … Pollack, S. (2004). Social functioning in children with ADHD treated with long-term methylphenidate and multimodal psychosocial treatment. *Journal of the American Academy of Child & Adolescent Psychiatry, 43*(7), 820–829.

American Psychiatric Association. (2013). *Diagnostic and statistical manual of mental disorders* (5th ed.). Washington, DC: Author.

Antshel, K. M. (2015). Psychosocial interventions in attention-deficit/hyperactivity disorder: Update. *Child and Adolescent Psychiatric Clinics of North America, 24*(1), 79–97.

Barkley, R. A. (Ed.). (2014). *Attention-deficit hyperactivity disorder: A handbook for diagnosis and treatment.* New York, NY: Guilford.

Bennett, C., Barlow, J., Huband, N., Smailagic, N., & Roloff, V. (2013). Group-based parenting programs for improving parenting and psychosocial functioning: A systematic review. *Journal of the Society for Social Work and Research, 4*(4), 300–332. doi:10.5243/jsswr.2013.20.

Biederman, J., Faraone, S. V., & Monuteaux, M. C. (2002). Differential effect of environmental adversity by gender: Rutter's Index of adversity in a group of boys and girls with and without ADHD. *American Journal of Psychiatry, 158*, 1556–1562.

Corman, C. L., & Trevino, E. (2009). *Eukee the jumpy jumpy elephant*. Plantation FL: Specialty Press, ADD Warehouse. Retrieved from the ADD Warehouse: http://www.addwarehouse.com/shopsite_sc/store/html/index.html

Cortese, S., Holtmann, M., Banaschewski, T., Buitelaar, J., Coghill, D., Danckaerts, M., ... Sergeant, J. (2013). Practitioner review: Current best practice in the management of adverse events during treatment with ADHD medications in children and adolescents. *Journal of Child Psychology and Psychiatry, 54*(3), 227–246.

Danckaerts, M., Sonuga-Barke, E. J., Banaschewski, T., Buitelaar, J., Döpfner, M., Hollis, C., ... Coghill, D. (2010). The quality of life of children with attention deficit/hyperactivity disorder: A systematic review. *European Child & Adolescent Psychiatry, 19*(2), 83–105. doi: 10.1007/s00787-009-0046-3/.

Dulcan, M. and the AACAP Work Group on Quality Issues. (1997). Practice parameters for the assessment and treatment of children, adolescents, and adults with attention-deficit/hyperactivity disorder. *Journal of the American Academy of Child & Adolescent Psychiatry, 36*(10 Suppl), 85S–121S.

Galvin, M. (2001). *Otto learns about his medicine: A story about medication for children with ADHD* (3rd ed.). Washington, DC: American Psychological Association/Magination Press.

Larson, K., Russ, S. A., Kahn, R. S., & Halfon, N. (2011). Patterns of comorbidity, functioning, and service use for US children with ADHD, 2007. *Pediatrics, 127*(3), 462–470. doi:10.1542/peds.2010-0165.

Molina, B. S., Hinshaw, S. P., Swanson, J. M., Arnold, L. E., Vitiello, B., Jensen, P. S., ... MTA Cooperative Group. (2009). The MTA at 8 years: Prospective follow-up of children treated for combined-type ADHD in a multisite study. *Journal of the American Academy of Child & Adolescent Psychiatry, 48*(5), 484–500.

Moss, D. (2006). *Shelley the hyperactive turtle*. Bethesda, MD: Woodbine House.

MTA Cooperative Group. (1999). A 14-month randomized clinical trial of treatment strategies for attention-deficit/hyperactivity disorder. *Archives of General Psychiatry, 56*(12), 1073–1086.

MTA Cooperative Group. (2004a). National Institute of Mental Health Multimodal Treatment Study of ADHD follow-up: 24-month outcomes of treatment strategies for attention-deficit/hyperactivity disorder. *Pediatrics, 113*(4), 754–761.

MTA Cooperative Group. (2004b). National Institute of Mental Health multimodal treatment study of ADHD follow-up: Changes in effectiveness and growth after the end of treatment. *Pediatrics, 113*, 762–769.

Pfiffner, L. J., Hinshaw, S. P., Owens, E., Zalecki, C., Kaiser, N. M., Villodas, M., & McBurnett, K. (2014). A two-site randomized clinical trial of integrated psychosocial treatment for ADHD-inattentive type. *Journal of Consulting and Clinical Psychology, 82*(6), 1115–1127. doi: 10.1037/a0036887.

Pliszka, S., & AACAP Work Group on Quality Issues. (2007). Practice parameter for the assessment and treatment of children and adolescents with attention-deficit/hyperactivity disorder. *Journal of the American Academy of Child & Adolescent Psychiatry, 46*(7), 894–921.

Quinn, P. O., & Stern, J. M. (2008). *Putting on the brakes: Understanding and taking control of your ADD or ADHD* (2nd ed.). Washington, DC: American Psychological Association/Magination Press.

Quinn, P. O., & Stern, J. M. (2009). *Putting on the brakes activity book for kids with ADD or ADHD*. Washington, DC: American Psychological Association/Magination Press.

Tamm, L., Nakonezny, P. A., & Hughes, C. W. (2014). An open trial of a metacognitive executive function training for young children with ADHD. *Journal of Attention Disorders, 18*(6), 551–559. doi:10.1177/1087054712445782.

Theule, J., Wiener, J., Tannock, R., & Jenkins, J. M. (2013). Parenting stress in families of children with ADHD: A meta-analysis. *Journal of Emotional and Behavioral Disorders, 21*(1), 3–17.

Watson, S. M. R., Richels, C., Michalek, A. P., & Raymer, A. (2015). Psychosocial treatments for ADHD: A systematic appraisal of the evidence. *Journal of Attention Disorders, 19*(1), 3–10.

Wolraich, M. L., Lambert, E. W., Baumgaertel, A., Garcia-Tornel, S., Feurer, I. D., Bickman, L., & Doffing, M. A. (2003). Teachers' screening for attention deficit/hyperactivity disorder: Comparing multinational samples on teacher ratings of ADHD. *Journal of Abnormal Child Psychology, 31*(4), 445–455.

Wolraich, M. L., Lambert, W., Doffing, M. A., Bickman, L., Simmons, T., & Worley, K. (2003). Psychometric properties of the Vanderbilt ADHD diagnostic parent rating scale in a referred population. *Journal of Pediatric Psychology, 28*(8), 559–568.

Wolraich, M. L., Lambert, E. W., Bickman, L., Simmons, T., Doffing, M. A., & Worley, K. A. (2004). Assessing the impact of parent and teacher agreement on diagnosing attention-deficit hyperactivity disorder. *Journal of Developmental & Behavioral Pediatrics, 25*(1), 41–47.

Chapter 11
Conclusion

Introduction

In this textbook, issues related to diagnosis, prevalence, assessment, management, and evidence-based interventions for children's health and mental health problems were reviewed. In addition to specific health problems, coping with pain was reviewed in a separate chapter, as this is a cross-cutting problem for children with many types of chronic illnesses. Information in the first chapter on the development of educational plans to solidify school planning for children provided important information for health professionals. Some children may experience cognitive delays or learning problems, and thus may benefit from receiving evaluation of their intellectual and academic achievement. Should discrepancies indicative of delays be discovered in either of the aforementioned areas, then children may benefit from the development of an Individual Education Program or Section 504 Plan to ensure that academic and social–emotional needs are met, as well as ensure regular evaluation of school functioning.

Children with Chronic Illnesses

Children with chronic illnesses and their families often gain significant knowledge from health education about the course and management of the child's chronic illness. Health problems for children can pose serious stress for the child and his or her family. Although, many children still function very well, and experience few problems, despite experiencing serious illnesses. Parents may not be able to "hear" information about their child's diagnosis and its impact, immediately after receiving the diagnosis. They may benefit from meeting with a health educator to discuss their child's diagnosis. The first year after the diagnosis can be a challenging period, and a time of adjustment, for children, parents, siblings, and extended family members.

© Springer International Publishing Switzerland 2016
L. Nabors, *Medical and Mental Health During Childhood*, Springer
Series on Child and Family Studies, DOI 10.1007/978-3-319-31117-3_11

Referral to a health educator for education and support may be a first step in empowering the child and family. Should significant mental health problems arise, or if family members are suffering from significant distress, then referral to a pediatric psychologist or child health psychologist should be considered. Children with chronic illnesses and their families may suffer from trauma related to the children's conditions, and health professionals should be familiar with grief and trauma reactions in children, parents, and immediate family members.

Some interventions are cross-cutting for children with different health conditions, such as using positive thinking and positive self-talk. Lessons to promote positive thinking and self-talk should be tailored to the individual needs of the child. A child with a chronic illness may need encouragement and information about social skills to interact more with children his or her age. If a great deal of time at school is missed due to illness, then the child would benefit from meetings between members of the medical team and school staff to ensure that school re-entry and re-integration goes on smoothly. In fact, developing a written plan for school re-entry and re-integration, allowing time to catch up and complete homework and assignments, plans for the child to return for a shorter day, and then moving to a fuller day at school, may be advantageous if a child is experiencing fatigue or problems with attention, memory, and organizational skills.

Other strategies that seemed to "commonly" apply to working with children with chronic illnesses were to have expertise in helping children adhere to medical regimens as well as having expertise in calming and relaxation strategies. In terms of adherence, health professionals need to have skills for teaching children and parents to monitor and record their child's progress in taking medications and following other steps of the child's medical regimen. Self-monitoring charts, to ensure that medications are taken as prescribed and to track diet and exercise behaviors are helpful. Having charts where the child can record pain or feelings about his or her illness can also provide the health professional with a window on how the child is feeling as he or she copes with his or her chronic illness. Parents and children may benefit from peer support and mentoring from children and parents who have "been there" and have experienced similar situations. Finally, teaching children to have a positive outlook and problem-solve and work with the medical team can build strengths and positive functioning for children. A problem-solving approach to the illness can be a significant positive factor in enhancing disease management, child coping, and quality of life. An emotion-based, avoidant coping style may not be a positive coping style for children. If health coaching does not move the child toward a more positive stance, then referral for mental health counseling, especially if the child is experiencing significant depression and anxiety, may be warranted.

Children with Mental Health Problems

In addition to a review of chronic illnesses for children, information on mental health problems for children was reviewed. Two main categories of mental health problems, internalizing problems, which involve worried, sad and anxious feelings, and externalizing problems, which may involve acting out and behavior problems, were reviewed. Internalizing problems are difficult for children, with anxiety being the most common internalizing issue for children. Some of the Cognitive Behavioral Therapy strategies described in the chapter focusing on anxiety disorders can be helpful for children with other types of mental health problems because they can help the child to stop and relax. If the child can stop and reset his or her system, then he or she may be more open to engaging in steps of problem-solving to think of a more productive behavior. For example, relaxation exercises, such as deep, slow breathing or making tight fists to squeeze out strong feelings can be tools to stop and reset one's system. Challenging negative thinking, such as anxious thoughts, can help a child realize that he or she can stop a negative cycle of thinking and make a positive change, improving his or her behavioral and emotional functioning. Teaching a child to use logic to work through and reshape negative thinking (such as thoughts that are anxiety-provoking, aggressive, or distressing) can assist a child in stopping a negative thinking pattern and using logical thinking and problem-solving to "think him- or herself into a new, positive way of acting."

Symptoms of worry and concern may limit a child's opportunities to have fun and play, which are primary avenues for learning and growing for children. Children's play, where they might typically describe themselves as having fun, is in actuality their learning ground, and if problems related to having a mental health disorder become more severe, then these symptoms can impede the child's play and subsequent social and emotional development. Similarly, externalizing problems can impede typical development for children. Externalizing problems or mental health issues are those that involve more acting out types of behaviors, such as being "off-task" or not being able to complete instructions and activities in the classroom, negative or aggressive behaviors, or impulsive behaviors (e.g., having difficulty remaining seated, impulsive or oppositional behaviors). We discussed attention problems and conduct problems as primary externalizing behavior problems. Children with externalizing problems can benefit from a very structured environment where there are clear cues for appropriate actions and a clear reward system for appropriate behaviors. If the child's behavior is very disruptive or the child is having difficulty following rules for appropriate behaviors, then clear consequences for negative behaviors can be helpful in setting boundaries for appropriate behavior.

For young children, it is important to involve their parents in treatment to improve emotional and behavioral functioning. Parents can be engaged to help build the child's self-esteem by ensuring that the child is engaged in activities in which he or she has a keen interest. Being interested in something and becoming "good at it" or building skill proficiency can be a self-esteem booster for children. Appropriate praise for positive accomplishments and at times, reward charts, with prizes and clear steps to attain good behavior or avoid negative behaviors can be helpful for young children. Positives, in terms of praise and small rewards, can go a long way in turning around patterns of negative behaviors in children. If a child is exhibiting harmful, aggressive, or disruptive behaviors—and the use of choices for alternative behaviors, distraction, and rewards are not successful—then use of consequences can be considered. Perhaps one of the most useful consequences is a response cost.

A response cost can be used if a child engages in a negative behavior and experiences a loss of a privilege, such as staying up late on a Friday night. Behaviors that will earn a response cost should be described clearly to the child, during a calm period, so that the child has a good understanding of what is expected of him or her.

Children with mental health problems also may benefit from social skills training. They may need to learn how to engage in turn-taking in conversations with peers and learn skills for entering play with peers. They may need to learn to share toys and use positive words when interacting with peers. As a result of social skill deficits, children can benefit from joining social skill groups, which may be offered in school settings. Children with externalizing problems benefit from learning to take another child's or adult's perspective. Children may need extra practice at learning steps to "stop and think" and consider other people's feelings as well as the possible ramifications of their behaviors before they act. Children with behavior problems may need to practice and be prompted to think of other people's feelings until they become more skilled at thinking about how others feel.

Problem-solving is a key skill for children. A step-by-step thinking process is important to review, so that children have a concrete plan for stopping to think and review ideas for appropriate behaviors. Some steps for teaching problem-solving can be remembered using the "STEPS" acronym, which was developed by the author of this textbook. The idea behind STEPS is that the child needs to actively take action or steps to solve a problem. The "S" stands for "seeing a problem" and this means that the child needs to identify that a problem exists. The health educator can help the child learn to identify things that are problems or barriers to positive functioning in his or her life. After the child sees a problem, then he or she must identify a strategy to make the problem better and "try" the strategy. This is the "T" step in STEPS. The health professional needs to teach the child (and his or her parents) many types of problem-solving strategies over a series of visits. Strategies are tailored to the child's problem areas, such as learning to take turns in conversations, use words to express feelings rather than yelling, or learning to relax rather than becoming angry and anxious. The child needs to take responsibility for generating and trying a strategy and child initiative and effort should be stressed as key components of becoming a positive problem-solver.

The next letter in STEPS is "E," which stands for evaluation or examining (put an eye on the problem to check how it is going) how things are going. After the child tries a positive strategy, then he or she needs to check and see if the strategy is working. A "working" strategy will help the child resolve a problem situation in a positive way. The child must evaluate whether the situation has improved in a positive way. Questions to ask are: "Has the situation improved?" or "Are things calm?" Other questions might include whether the child or others are still feeling angry or upset in some way. Next, is the "P" another critical part of the STEPS approach. For the "P" activity the child needs to praise him or herself for being a problem-solver. This builds self-esteem and the child's self-efficacy for engaging in problem-solving. The final letter is "S." The "S" stands for "see the problem again." This means that the child takes another look at the original problem to determine if it went away or is reduced in scope. The child then needs to make a determination about whether another STEPS cycle is needed. The health professional needs to teach the child that problem-solving is an iterative process such that, "if you don't succeed, try and try again." Many times when the child is trying to learn problem-solving it is beneficial to engage parents in the problem-solving activities and use a reward chart for praising and rewarding the child for working on problem-solving.

When children with mental health problems experience co-occurring or comorbid learning problems, they can benefit from assessment of their intellectual and achievement functioning. Children with social and emotional problems (i.e., internalizing and externalizing mental health diagnoses) also can benefit from Section 504 plans or Individual Education Programs if behavioral, emotional, and social problems significantly interfere with their academic performance. In the same fashion, if they have co-occurring learning problems, such school-based plans are necessary. Consultation with the school psychologist and the special education team at the child's school will assist in jump-starting an evaluation process.

Children Learn Skills Over Time, with Practice

Children typically need time, repeated instruction, and practice to learn new ways of thinking about their behavior and new ways of acting. There may be "windows of readiness" or times when they are more open to learning new skills for changing negative ways of thinking or behaving. Similarly, for children with chronic illnesses, there may be optimal times, given their attitudes and other life factors, for teaching a child to adhere to his or her medical regimen or perhaps take a greater role in self-management of his or her illness. Thus, health educators need to consider a child's readiness and his or her stage of development when teaching a child new skills. In terms of developmental stage, it is very important to ensure that teaching is developmentally appropriate or at the right level for the child. The teaching has to be at a level where the child can understand and learn new skills. In a similar way, health educators need to be able to meet the child's parents or caregivers wherever they are, in order to teach and support them. A child's and family's needs, skills, and openness to education will evolve over time and the health educator needs to be flexible and ready to help when needed.

Systems Approach

The systems in which a child is involved impact his or her functioning. As mentioned in Chap. 1, the child is embedded in a family, school, neighborhood, and larger community. These systems or contexts can impact a child's development, learning, and reactions. Those systems closer to the child, such as the family and school, may have the most impact on the child. Key players in those systems, such as parents and teachers, are key sources of information about the child's functioning. The health educator should interview parents and teachers to obtain and monitor child progress. A next step is to determine how the child's health or mental health problem is impacting his or her functioning. After assessing the child's capabilities, the health educator can make a determination of whether the parents (caregivers) or teachers can help implement interventions to assist the child in improving his or her functioning.

Another definition of context is the setting in which the child finds him- or herself. The setting can be a key tool in creating change for a child. Changing the child's seat in the classroom, for example, by moving it closer to the teacher, can make a difference for a child with attention problems and difficulties with concentration. Teaching parents to ensure that the child has enough sleep can make a world of difference in the child's behaviors. Teaching parents to use rewards for positive behaviors and ignore negative behaviors, can help a child turn around behaviors. Moreover, this type of discipline can be positive in that the child is not exposed to aggressive behavior, such as when harsh and inconsistent consequences, such as yelling, threats with no follow-through, and hostile or angry spanking is used by the parent. Reducing noise and giving transition warnings, with visual cards using a list of words or pictures to let a child know his or her schedule, are contextual changes that can help a child with Autism Spectrum Disorders in the school setting. The preceding context changes are examples of ways in which setting or environmental changes can help a child achieve better behavioral functioning, which can improve emotional functioning as well.

As mentioned in Chap. 1, children are embedded in key systems in their lives. These systems are key contexts through which a child's development unfolds. Perhaps the closest in proximity are the family, with parental, sibling, and extended family influences, and school influences. Parents and schools were a focus of chapters addressing key health and mental health problems for children. Along the same vein, siblings and extended family are key players in many children's development. They should be involved in efforts to support the child. Moreover, siblings and extended family may need to be included in sessions to educate the child and parents about health and mental health problems. These sessions typically involve skill building and developing coping strategies. Extended family and siblings should be included in sessions whenever their involvement can build a better environment for the child.

Broader systems involve coaches and leaders in extracurricular activities for the child as well as friends and their parents. These stakeholders, if they are key players for the child, may need to be educated about the child's condition and learn about ways that they can support the child. For example, if a child has arthritis or diabetes, coaches and band leaders may need education about allowing the child breaks to rest if in pain (a child with arthritis) or breaks to test blood sugar levels (if the child has diabetes). These activity leaders may need education about how to explain a child's condition to other children involved in the activity. It may be beneficial for the health educator to attend a group meeting (of the children involved in the

Table 11.1 Key systems, besides family and school, in children's lives

System	How the system can influence a child
Coach and team	The terms "coach" and "team" broadly refer to leaders of recreational or extracurricular activities and other children involved in the activity. These key players influence a child's self-esteem, feelings of self-efficacy, and these activities allow the child to develop social skills and other skills such as motor abilities, athletic skills, musical abilities, leadership skills, etc.
Neighborhood play	Children play with a variety of peers and experience many adult influences in their neighborhoods. Play allows a child to interact with peers, build a sense of efficacy as well as learn sharing and give and take in social interactions. Through play a child begins to build life experience while undertaking many different roles
Extended family	Extended family can impact parent behaviors and the reciprocity between the parent and child can heavily influence child functioning. Extended family can play key mentoring roles—for example, when parents have to work or when children develop special relationships with extended family (e.g., grandparents), which allow them to become role models
Economic environment	The economic environment in the neighborhood or home can influence child development. If finances are scarce at home, family stress and parent distress can influence a child's outlook on life and their interactions with parents. In an impoverished neighborhood environment, children can experience violence and other negative influences (e.g., gang influences, drugs)
Political structures	The political structures in the child's environment, such as in the school, their neighborhood, and their country can impact what a child learns about civil rights, violence, and a host of other factors

Note: These are a few examples of systems that can influence a child. Others might be religion, parent–work environment, siblings' friends, etc.

activity) and explain ways to support and interact with the child. The environment also may need to be modified to foster the inclusion of the child with a special health or mental health care need. For instance, if a child was in a wheelchair and was in band, chairs may need to be situated so that the child can maneuver his or her wheelchair into position. If a child had Attention-Deficit/Hyperactivity Disorder, the school nurse and school staff will need to make efforts to ensure that the child receives medication in a private area and that undue attention is not drawn to the child when he or she has to leave the classroom to take medication. There are many other "systems" examples and some of these are outlined in Table 11.1.

Support for the Child and Family

Support for the child and family is a key intervention across a myriad of health and mental health conditions. The child benefits from support of peers and adults. Instrumental support occurs when tangible supports are put in place for the child, such as having an extra set of textbooks for the child to have at home or having a teacher go to the hospital to go over homework for a child who has a chronic illness. Tangible or instrumental support for a child with a mental health problem can be a reward chart, with behavioral expectations clearly specified, with rewards indicated for a specific number of positive behaviors. To illustrate, a child with a tendency to be aggressive on the playground could have a playground chart, with specific behaviors such as sharing, joining in with others, and saying positive things to peers clearly described. If the child exhibited positive behaviors twice per playground outing, then he or she could receive a small prize. The rewards could become harder to obtain as the child masters higher levels of positive behaviors.

Children with chronic illnesses may receive social support from peers with the same illnesses when they attend a summer camp with children with the same type of illness. Alternately, they can receive social support from peer groups at a local children's hospital. Friends can provide support, and a health educator can help maximize peer support by educating peers about the condition and teaching peers how to interact with and support the child. Children with mental health problems can receive social support in social skills groups at school, from peer buddies, or from children they befriend in extracurricular activities. Health educators should be aware of support needs and be proactive in planning ways to support children with health and mental health problems.

Similarly, parents of children with health or mental health problems benefit from support. They benefit from support of parents, who can also serve as mentors, of children with similar problems. Support from the medical team, counselor, or child psychiatrist is critical in providing parents with confidence and self-efficacy. Health educators should be familiar with how to support parents as they grieve the loss of their child's "free and easy childhood years" if the child must struggle with a health or mental health problem. If a child has a serious illness understanding parents' feelings (denial, grief, anger, sadness, and a wealth of other feelings) can help support them. Health educators can play a key role in educating parents about illness, finding support groups or mentors, and being a healing presence as the parent copes with grief because his or her child is faced with a significant problem.

Siblings

Brothers and sisters influence a child's development. Interactions between siblings can enhance a child's coping with a chronic illness or mental health problem. Their support can be a vital uplift. For instance, at a local Ronald McDonald House, where this author volunteers, brothers and sisters provide support by developing blogs or Facebook pages where the child with the illness can reach out to extended family and be contacted by extended family. The child can find support from others in his or her community and make new friends through his or her blog or Facebook page. This can be a way to reach out and be in community with others. It is noteworthy, however, that parents should remain active in their child's life by monitoring blogs and Facebook pages to make sure that communications are positive.

Siblings can face confusion when a brother or sister faces a serious health or mental health problem. They can lack understanding of what is happening and feel "in the dark" about what is going on with their brother or sister. The sibling also could feel guilty because they do not have any type of problem, while their brother or sister must face a serious problem. It may be likely that the sibling could feel "left out" and miss parental attention, as the parent may need to extend extra support, time, and care to help a child with a health or mental health problem. The sibling can feel depressed and isolated. Alternately, the sibling could "act out" and exhibit behavioral problems to gain attention and time from the parent and other family members. Health educators can play a role in the education of siblings about a brother or sister's medical condition and helping them to understand how problem affects their brother's or sister's life. It may be necessary to refer siblings for counseling should they be having significant difficulty adjusting to their brother's or sister's condition. Health educators should monitor sibling engagement in meaningful activities. A sibling can be "forgotten" when a parent has to focus attention on a child with a serious problem. Siblings still need to be involved, to the extent possible, in activities, because involvement in activities can help them learn new skills, feel a sense of personal achievement, build self-esteem, and make friendships that will support their growth and development.

Children Are Agents in Their Own Development

Children are active in constructing their own development. They are active in constructing their own personalities. They influence their parents, just as their parents (and for that matter, other key adults in their lives) influence them. Children learn to think and can make decisions early. Their moods and their behaviors shape parent reactions and the reactions of other key players' in their lives. The child changes over time as well. As the child develops, and different experiences in his or her life unfold, the child's own views and agency shape experiences. Hence, there is a cyclical interaction between the child's own personality and wishes and what occurs in the child's life that shapes the child's view of him- or herself and the world. Figure 11.1 illustrates the reciprocity between the child and experience, with the child having a key role as an agent in his or her development over time.

Figure 11.1 is complex, yet it is surely missing some of the key factors that may interact and influence some children's lives. Throughout all that happens to the child, however, the child's own temperament or personality has an influence on his or her development. The child is embedded in settings, historical context, and other factors that interact to influence his or her development. These notions harken back to previous theoretical orientations, such as that of Urie Bronfenbrenner (1979, 1989), who proposed that children are active in their development, but are impacted by change over time and other systems in their lives. Bronfenbrenner developed Ecological Systems Theory, positing that children were embedded in systems, such as the family, neighborhood, country, etc. that played a key role in influencing their

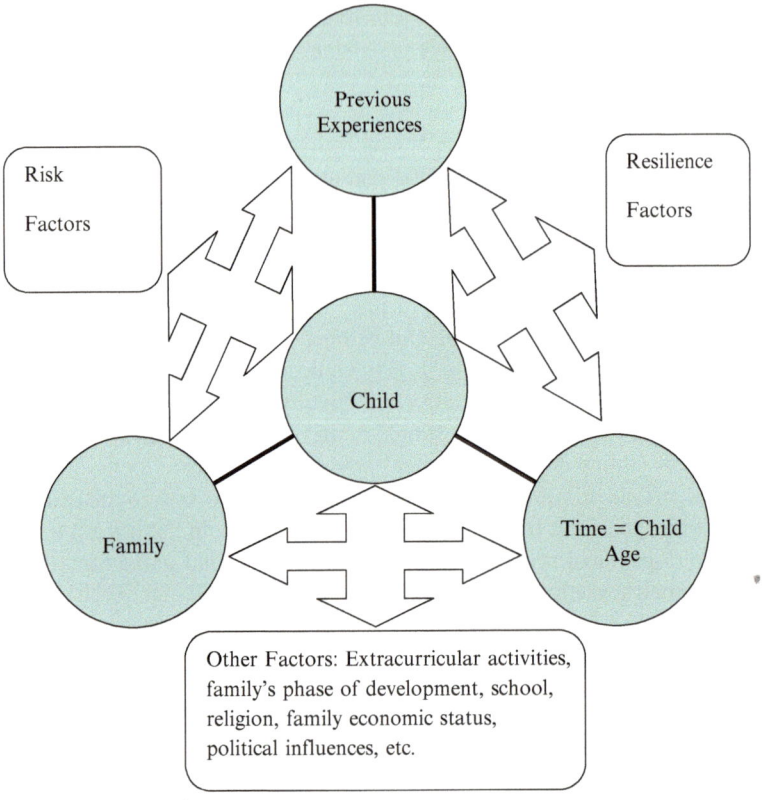

Fig. 11.1 Children as agents in their own development—within a multi-determined world

development over the course of their lives. Systems that are distant from the child, such as the parents' work environment could also influence his or her development. If a mother or father had a bad work environment, and came home upset every evening, this removed setting could have a negative impact on the child through his or her interactions with an "upset" parent. Another famous theorist, Albert Bandura (1978, 1986) posited that behavior is reciprocally determined, and is influenced by the person, what has happened in previous situations, as well as other environmental factors. Bandura's theory of reciprocal determinism opened exploration into the interaction of personal factors, such as will and motivation, the valence of what happened in past experiences for the person (either good or bad outcomes), and the influence of factors inherent in the environment, as being critical to influencing behavior and development.

Moreover, the phase of development for the child (e.g., child age) and the family (where the family is in its development as a unit) will influence the child's development. To illustrate, a family may be in emotional turmoil because parents are getting a divorce, which impacts the emotional development and functioning of the entire family. Divorce may have a very strong impact on children in the preschool years.

Historical impacts, such as war or natural disaster can also impact a child's developmental course. The boxes in Fig. 11.1 represent factors that can impact child development. The bi-directional arrows reflect the reciprocal influence of the child and key factors in his or her environment, past experiences, and settings (contexts) that also may interact with the child's own beliefs and temperament to influence his or her developmental trajectory.

The interactions between the child, significant others in his or her life, time in the child's life, and phase of development for the child and family are very complex. These factors are multidimensional and can have differential impacts on each other. It may be impossible to figure out how much of which factor contributed to child functioning. The health educator needs to take a careful history and understand all of the factors that impact a child, how his or her parents and significant others influence the child, and how life events which occur in different settings influence the child's functioning. When taking a careful history and understanding all the factors contributing to a child's functioning, the health educator has a chance to develop a comprehensive plan that considers the child's strengths and factors in the environment that would facilitate positive functioning for the child.

Risk and resilience factors impact all aspects of a child's development (see Fig. 11.1). If the model were three-dimensional and if it was moving, then these key factors would always be at play. They interact with all factors within the child and those in the child's environment. Risk and resilience factors may be at the level of the child, family, settings in the child's life (extracurricular activities, neighborhood, religion), in historical factors (heroes that touch the child's life during times of tragedy, such as war or natural disasters). These factors impact how the child perceives experiences in his or her life. For instance, believing in oneself and having confidence is a resilience factor. A risk factor, inherent to the child's character, may be having a personality that is prone toward risk-taking behaviors. A resilience factor in the family might be a tendency to stick together in the face of adversity, whereas divorce in the family might be a risk factor. An upturn in the economy might be a resilience factor, if an unemployed parent gets a job. A strong mentor for an after-school activity might be another resilience factor.

When the health educator is developing plans to enhance child functioning, determining ways to maximize the impact of resilience factors and minimize the effects of risk factors are critical to developing successful plans to enhance child functioning. Teaching the child how to capitalize on positives in his or her world and move toward a positive developmental trajectory, maximizing resilient functioning, is a very active view of child agency. The health educator needs to take into consideration a child's overall health and its role in improving child agency. Making sure a child has a good sense of self, gets enough rest, and eats healthy food are key factors in ensuring that the child can be active in determining a positive outcome for him- or herself. In fact, good child health and mental health may be cornerstones to child agency and positive development. As shown in Fig. 11.1, the child is in the center of many factors that shape his or her life. The child will have some agency in directing and influencing his or her world. This figure depicts many avenues for hope as there are many points of intervention to develop interventions to bring positive factors to bear in improving a child's life.

Summary

This final chapter has offered an opportunity to present some critical ideas about the child and his or her role in shaping development. Moreover, information about environmental factors and other influences on a child's development, such as child stage of development and family stage of development, have been explored. Key factors impacting the child, such as diagnosis, child personality, family, school, and neighborhood contexts, and risk and resilience factors, have been presented as crucial variables influencing the child. The health educator, when understanding that factors can change and the child can be active in influencing change, has a very positive role to play in designing intervention and care plans to support the child. Indeed, the future can be viewed as very bright for children as there are many avenues and directions for developing positive movement toward growth! Supporting the child to improve his or her self-confidence and beliefs in his or her ability to produce change is a positive beginning in any plan of care. Supporting family growth and promoting the development of resilience factors and reducing risk for the child and family are continual goals in improving child wellness and health. As such, similar to the child, health educators could conceive of their role as active agents in search of and promoting positive change through environmental and personal interventions that enhance coping of the child and his or her family.

Reducing barriers to good health and mental healthcare and improving child access to positive factors, such as involvement in after-school activities and activities with friends, are valuable actions to facilitate positives for the child. Ensuring that child wellness and growth through healthy eating, exercise, positive mental health and stress reduction are key factors to improving child functioning. Promoting access to an appropriate education and positive family and social environment are other system level goals to enhance child wellness and growth. Understanding the risks children face (through research and clinical experience), and working to improve their resilience and positive factors in their environments, affords opportunities for health educators to change children's lives for the better. In closing, it is hoped that reading this book has provided new information and encouragement for students to work in the field to improve the lives of children and their families.

Exercises/Review Questions

1. Discuss your ideas for interventions to promote feelings of self-efficacy for children with chronic illnesses or mental health problems. Feel free to browse the internet for creative ideas.
2. Discuss ways you would promote problem-solving skills for children with mental health problems.
3. Some key systems are the school and neighborhood. How do these two contexts influence development for a child with a chronic illness or a child with a mental health problem?
4. Child stage of development (e.g., being in early childhood versus high school) impacts a child's functioning and world view. Similarly, family stage of development can impact child and family functioning. Thus, compare and contrast how

a family with several very young children might interact with a child with oppositional behaviors versus a family with much older children, where parents are about to face an empty nest.

5. Figure 11.1 presents a complex model of factors effecting child agency. Do you agree with the concepts in this model? Why or why not? What does your own model of child agency and development look like? What factors are key to influencing child growth and wellness in your personal model?

Key Concepts

STEPS model of problem-solving

Systems approach

Reciprocal influence of different developmental factors on each other

Albert Bandura (Reciprocal Determinism)

Urie Bronfenbrenner (Ecological Systems Theory)

Child agency

Risk Factors

Resilience Factors

References

Bandura, A. (1978). The self system in reciprocal determinism. *American Psychologist, 33*(4), 344–358.

Bandura, A. (1986). *Social foundations of thought and action: A social cognitive theory*. Englewood Cliffs, NJ: Prentice Hall.

Bronfenbrenner, U. (1979). *The ecology of human development: Experiments by nature and design*. Cambridge, MA: Harvard University Press.

Bronfenbrenner, U. (1989). Ecological systems theory. *Annals of Child Development, 6*, 187–249.

ERRATUM

Chapter 8
Depression

© Springer International Publishing Switzerland 2016
L. Nabors, *Medical and Mental Health During Childhood*, Springer
Series on Child and Family Studies, DOI 10.1007/978-3-319-31117-3_8

DOI 10.1007/978-3-319-31117-3_12

The author's name and affiliation in the original chapter entitled, "Depression", is incorrectly stated.

For chapter 8, the author's name and affiliation should read as follows:

Ashley Merianos, Ph.D.
Health Promotion and Education, School of Human Services,
College of Education, Criminal Justice and Human Services
University of Cincinnati, Cincinnati, OH, USA

The online version of the original chapter can be found at
http://dx.doi.org/10.1007/978-3-319-31117-3_8

© Springer International Publishing Switzerland 2016
L. Nabors, *Medical and Mental Health During Childhood*, Springer
Series on Child and Family Studies, DOI 10.1007/978-3-319-31117-3_12

Index

© Springer International Publishing Switzerland 2016
L. Nabors, *Medical and Mental Health During Childhood*, Springer
Series on Child and Family Studies, DOI 10.1007/978-3-319-31117-3